MAHARISHI AYURVEDA AND VEDIC TECHNOLOGY

Creating Ideal Health for the Individual and World

ALSO BY ROBERT KEITH WALLACE

An Introduction to Transcendental Meditation (with Lincoln Norton)

Transcendental Meditation (Physiology of Consciousness: Part 1)

The Neurophysiology of Enlightenment

Dharma Parenting (with Fred Travis)

Dharma Health and Beauty (with Samantha Wallace)

MAHARISHI AYURVEDA AND VEDIC TECHNOLOGY

Creating Ideal Health for the Individual and World

Adapted and Updated from
The Physiology of Consciousness: Part 2

Robert Keith Wallace PhD

Dharma Publications

ISBN 978-0-9972207-3-5

Library of Congress Control Number: 2016932098

www.DharmaPublications.com

Dharma Publications, Fairfield, IA

Contents

TO
MAHARISHI MAHESH YOGI

Chapter 1

Ayurveda and Maharishi Ayurveda

A number of years ago I was invited to speak at a physicians' conference in Massachusetts. As I drove up the long driveway to the health center, surrounded by many acres of snowy woods, I felt pleased to be in New England once again. Although I was born in California, my real roots are in New England, where I spent years as a youth and where most of my relatives still live.

New England is also one source of my deep interest in health and human physiology. My grandfather, who had a strong influence on all my family, was a pioneer in his field, a surgeon who graduated from Harvard Medical School, worked with the Mayo brothers, and was a founding member of the New England Surgical Society. After performing several historic operations he established his own hospital in Fall River, Massachusetts. To me he represents the good that modern medicine stands for.

So it was natural for me in this New England setting to think of how my grandfather might have regarded Maharishi

Ayurveda and Vedic Technology and their applications to health. I am sure that he, like most physicians, would have thought it strange at first to go back in time and restore an ancient tradition of knowledge in order to help modern medicine become more complete and effective. However, I think that if he could have been there at the conference and heard about the numerous research studies and the full range of medical strategies available, he would have been keenly interested.

Ayurveda and Maharishi Ayurveda

Ayurveda is an ancient and comprehensive system of natural health, considered to be the grandfather of all traditional medical systems. The term Ayurveda comes from two Sanskrit words, *ayus*, meaning "life" or "lifespan," and *Veda*, meaning "knowledge" or "science." Ayurveda may be translated as "the science of life," or, more specifically, "the science of lifespan." Ayurveda offers knowledge about every aspect of life and health. However, due to India's history of political turbulence, over hundreds of years, this knowledge became fragmented; much was forgotten, and the rest known only to a few experts.

Today, not many people think of India as a source of new information about health. There is no question that India has severe health problems and needs solutions, starting with the teaching of basic personal hygiene in the villages, and extending to the introduction of complete approaches of health in order to deal with the alarming rate of the new incidence of modern stress-related disease, especially in urban areas.

Yet India is the source of the knowledge of yoga and meditation, which are so popular among natural health enthusiasts. India's Vedic tradition is one of the oldest in the world, and only now are we even beginning to fathom its great wisdom. This is the tradition from which Ayurveda comes.

We might have heard about Ayurveda from some popular health TV show or magazine article, but it is still largely unknown to most medical professionals. Even though it has been used for thousands of years, acceptance in the West depends upon scientific research and controlled clinical trials.

Two examples in which the advances in modern medicine might help medical professionals to understand and better accept the programs of Ayurveda, are the new fields of personalized medicine and lifestyle medicine.

Personalized medicine identifies genetic and metabolic differences between individuals, and prescribes treatment programs based on unique identifiers. One of the benefits of this approach is that phyicians are able to determine how well a patient metabolizes a particular drug, and, therefore, can more precisely determine the ideal dose and minimize side effects.

Ayurveda is entirely based on a personalized system of medicine, which is time-tested over millenia, and is based on a profound analysis of individual body nature. Recent scientific studies, as we will discuss later, have shown that

Ayurveda's personalized body typing system has now been validated by modern research, using genetic and biochemical analysis.

Lifestyle medicine is another new field. It recognizes that many modern diseases, such as heart disease and diabetes, are caused by poor lifestyle and habits. The physician endeavors to prevent and cure disorders by modifying the patient's behavior through changes in diet, exercise, sleep, and stress management.

Ayurveda and other traditional systems of medicine have always placed significant importance on lifestyle in order to maintain ideal health. Ayurveda possesses remarkable techniques for detecting imbalances in the mind and body, and includes extensive recommendations for changing individual lifestyle in order to restore balance and prevent disease.

In addition to these trends in modern medicine, there are also a growing number of studies on the medicinal plants used in Ayurveda. In a later chapter, we will review some of these extraordinary findings.

One individual responsible for creating a huge interest in Ayurveda in the mid 1980s, and for reviving its effectiveness, is Maharishi Mahesh Yogi, founder of the Transcendental Meditation technique. It was Maharishi's genius to restore the consciousness aspect of Ayurveda. This is one of the main differences between Ayurveda and Maharishi Ayurveda. This precious knowledge was originally an integral part of Ayurveda, but over time became lost, abandoned, or misinterpreted. Maharishi re-introduced specific techniques to allow the individual to develop his own consciousness as the basis for a healthy physiology.

Once Maharishi had restored the consciousness aspect of Ayurveda, his next step was to work with the remaining leading experts of traditional Ayurveda to revive the completeness of this knowledge. When this great task was completed, lectures and symposia were held at leading research institutes and universities around the world, encouraging scientific research on all the various therapeutic strategies of Maharishi Ayurveda. In the United States, experts in Maharishi Ayurveda spoke to such prominent forums as the National Institutes of Health, Johns Hopkins Medical School, Yale Medical School, Harvard School of Public Health, and Massachusetts General Hospital. These presentations were received everywhere with great interest, and many studies have since been undertaken to investigate the programs of Maharishi Ayurveda.

Maharishi Ayurveda contains highly refined techniques for both the diagnosis and treatment of disease. These techniques are based on an understanding of the body as a network of intelligence, which is the microcosm of all nature. The most important of these is the Transcendental Meditation (or TM) technique.

The Transcendental Meditation Technique

TM is a simple and effortless mental technique that is practiced 20 minutes twice each day, sitting comfortably with the eyes closed. It involves no mood, belief, or special lifestyle—it simply allows the mind to settle inward, through quieter levels of thought, until one experience the most silent and peaceful level of one's own awareness.

Over 380 published studies have documented its effectiveness at improving both physical and mental health. The TM technique optimizes brain functioning allowing an individual to become more successful and fulfilled in activity. It provides an effective and natural means of dissolving deeply rooted stress and fatigue, and unfolds the full value of life.

A number of important studies have shown that TM reduces high blood pressure and cardiovascular disease. A statement from the American Heart Association concluded that the Transcendental Meditation technique is the only meditation practice that has been shown to lower blood pressure. One significant study found that African Americans with heart disease who practiced the Transcendental Meditation technique regularly were 48 % less likely to have a heart attack or stroke, or to die from other causes—as compared with African Americans who attended a health education class for more than five years. Researchers who conducted the study at the Medical College of Wisconsin in Milwaukee, reported that the more regularly the patients meditated, the longer their survival rate.

In terms of health utilization, several important studies have revealed that TM markedly reduces health care costs. In a five-year study on some two thousand individuals, meditators use medical and surgical health care services approximately one-half as often as other insurance users. In Québec, Canada, researchers compared the changes in physician costs for TM practitioners with non-practitioners over a five-year period. After the first year, the TM group's health care costs decreased 11%, and after five years their cumulative reduction was 28%. The TM patients required fewer referrals, resulting in lower medical expenses such as tests, prescription drugs, hospitalization, surgery, and other treatments.

One important psychological study on TM shows a significant decrease in levels of anxiety after starting TM, as compared to subjects practicing other relaxation techniques. Psychological studies on TM have also shown decreased neuroticism, depression, and aggression, with increased self-esteem, moral reasoning, and self-actualization. Studies also show that TM improves different aspects of student life—from improved academic performance and reduced anxiety, to increased energy level, self-esteem, tolerance, creativity, and intelligence.

The David Lynch Foundation has brought the Transcendental Meditation technique to over half a million school children in the United States, Brazil, Peru, Bolivia, Vietnam,

Nepal, Northern Ireland, Ghana, Kenya, Uganda, South Africa, and Israel. In addition, it has provided TM to veterans, and to female victims of domestic violence and abuse, to soldiers and refugees suffering from PTSD, prisoners, the homeless, and to American Indians—all with positive results.

TM is not a religion, philosophy, or lifestyle. Over six million people of all ages, cultures, and backgrounds practice this effortless and effective technique of meditation. To overcome our prejudices, we must understand that just because Transcendental Meditation comes from India, that doesn't make its application specific to that culture. The fact that Einstein, a German Jew, arrived at his famous theory of relativity while working at a patent office in Switzerland doesn't make his theory Swiss, German, or Jewish. In our age of science we are able to perceive principles of nature that transcend cultural boundaries and traditions.

Maharishi Health Centers

Maharishi created a plan to improve the health of the world. This plan includes the establishment of an integrative system of health, which combines the best of Ayurveda, the best of modern medicine, and the best of all other traditional systems of medicine. Maharishi's plan incorporates the creation of a network of Maharishi Health Centers to effectively prevent disease and reduce the burden of chronic disease, as well as the establishment of Maharishi Colleges of Perfect Health for the proper training of health professionals. It also includes the creation of scientific research institutes to study all systems of traditional medicine in order to determine the most effective treatment programs.

The entire world is in great need of a new system of medicine, one that encompasses both the modern technology of our age and the ancient understanding and technologies of health. Only by shifting our attention away from a totally disease-oriented approach and by recognizing the need for a preventive approach with a profound basis in knowledge and effective practices, will we be able to curb increasing health care costs. A better understanding of the fundamental principles that govern our mind and body will enable us to eliminate today's major killer-diseases and promote an ideal state of health for every person in the world.

Chapter 2

The Finest Layers of Our Physiology of Matter

I once escorted a distinguished physician and scientist—a woman responsible for the health care of several million people in her own country—through one of the first Maharishi Ayurveda centers in North America. After touring the facility she sat in on several interviews with patients. The first case she heard was that of a young woman named Anne, age thirty-two. Anne was having a regular checkup and reported some sleep disorders and indigestion.

After a physical examination that involved both a routine Western and more specialized Ayurvedic examination, the clinic's doctor told her that she had been experiencing some unusual anger for the last three days. Anne had been perfectly calm throughout, with no physiological or psychological evidence of anger. She was visibly surprised and said, "Yes, I have been angry at several things lately. How did you know? Did my husband tell you?" "No," the doctor laughed, "no one told me. Anger is one of the primary symptoms of your particular body nature when there is a metabolic imbalance, and this imbalance is quite evident from your examination. I'm going to prescribe a few simple changes in diet and daily routine which will correct it."

After Anne had left the room, our visitor turned to the doctor in amazement. "How could you possibly determine that this woman has been angry for three days?" He explained that Anne's particular body nature was prone to the emotion of anger, and also that Anne's responses to a diagnostic questionnaire and her pulse diagnosis gave clear indications of certain imbalances. The visitor witnessed several such displays of diagnosis, and by the end of the visit she was both impressed and enthusiastic. I had no difficulty explaining the concept of Ayurvedic body typing and its great value in helping to cure and, more importantly, prevent disease.

The Fundamental Structure of Matter

One of the central concepts described in classical Ayurvedic texts is known as *Panchamahabhuta*. This describes how matter arises from consciousness. What is particularly interesting in this theory is the description of the finer layers of our physiology.

In this theory, the universe's origin is *avyakta*, "unmanifest"—the unmanifest unified field of pure consciousness. Arising from this field (the Self) are the various levels of the physiology of consciousness: ego, intellect, mind, and senses. These levels form the "anatomy" of consciousness. They are broad principles and structures of natural law at the foundation of everything in creation—the basis for the entire universe, which includes the human body.

As the laws of nature sequentially unfold through the self-interacting dynamics of pure consciousness, Maharishi explains how eventually the structures of natural law take on a concrete form, and consciousness gives rise to matter: Through sequential development consciousness unfolds itself into the value of matter; consciousness becomes matter. The Self becomes mind, and mind becomes matter. We see an analogy of this in modern physiology, when the DNA, which contains all the information necessary to create and maintain our body, transcribes and translates that knowledge into material proteins, which in turn structure the body systems. This transformation of the field of pure knowledge rising from DNA as the impulse of information in RNA, to RNA becoming protein and protein becoming the whole material system, is the description of consciousness becoming matter.

There is thus a transition point in the sequential unfoldment of natural law, at which the subjective physiology of consciousness gives rise to the objective physiology of matter. Maharishi explains that this is a self-referral process. He describes how this intimate and delicate connection between consciousness and matter takes place at the point when the subjective impulse of thought is becoming translated, through the DNA, into RNA and then into proteins:

> This transformation is sequential but always self-referral. It
> is like the airplane flying but always remaining self-referral

to the ground station through the radio. All the activities of DNA, RNA, protein, and the whole system are always self-referral. When a mosquito comes and immediately the hand moves, it is the DNA that orders, "Look here! The danger is coming, you get up." This performance is self-referral because consciousness, intelligence, is developing itself into different expressions of its own nature and there is continuity between matter and pure consciousness—the Self, the mind, and the body.

In this progression from Self to mind to body, we can look in finer detail at what happens at the transition point from subjectivity to objectivity. From the perspective of Panchamahabhuta theory in Maharishi Ayurveda, the finest level of matter in creation is described in terms of five basic constituents: *akasha* (space), *vayu* (air), *agni* (fire), *jal* (water), and *prithivi* (earth). Pancha means "five"; thus the term panchamahabhuta means "five elements." These five basic constituents have a subtle and a gross aspect. The subtle aspect is referred to as the five *tanmatras* and the gross aspect as the five *mahabhutas.* The five tanmatras are associated with the five senses. On the borderline between consciousness and matter, the senses are still within the subjective physiology of consciousness, and Maharishi explains that the tanmatras are the finest material expression of these five principles of nature:

> The tanmatras constitute the five basic realities, or essences, of the objects of the five senses of perception. They express themselves in the five elements which go to make up the objects of the senses and which provide the material basis of the entire objective universe. Thus the essence of sound

(shabda tanmatra) expresses itself in space, the essence of touch (sparsha tanmatra) in air, the essence of form (rupa tanmatra) in fire, the essence of taste (rasa tanmatra) in water, and the essence of smell (gandha tanmatra) in earth... The tanmatras mark the dividing line between the subjective and objective creation. In the process of evolution, . . . the subjective creation comes to an end and the objective creation begins. The tanmatras, forming as they do the basis of the five elements, lie in the grossest field of the subjective aspect of creation.

The five mahabhutas (akasha, vayu, etc.) are the same principles, found at a slightly more concrete level of the physiology of matter. Maharishi explains that they are the "elements out of which material creation is constituted"; the entire material creation evolves from these five fundamental elements. They are considered the building blocks from which matter arises.

In terms of our modern scientific understanding of the body, these concepts are perhaps more the concern of the most advanced and abstract areas of physics, having to do with the mechanics of nature that underlie biological functioning.

Dr. John Hagelin, one of the world's leading physicists in the area of unified quantum field theories, has interpreted the Panchamahabhuta theory in the terms of modern physics. Dr. Hagelin is also an expert in Maharishi Vedic Science and Technology, and in two articles, "Is Consciousness the Unified Field? A Field Theorist's Perspective," and "Restructuring Physics from its Foundation in Light of Maharishi Vedic Science," he outlines the discovery of the unified field and its relationship to consciousness. In his discussion he makes use not only of the latest knowledge of modern quantum physics, but also of "the very complete description of the unified field and its self-interacting dynamics provided by Vedic Science as formulated by Maharishi Mahesh Yogi." In discussing the elementary particles and forces of nature, Dr. Hagelin explains that Maharishi Vedic Science "provides a very natural and compact language of nature which is also based directly on the unified field."

In Dr. Hagelin's view, the transition from consciousness into matter in human life represents the junction point between the quantum mechanical and classical in the structure of the human physiology. He suggests that there is a distinct similarity between the five fundamental elements described in Maharishi Vedic Science and Technology, and the fundamental spin types of quantum physics (he refers to the five elements as tanmatras rather than mahabhutas to emphasize their subtlest value). He first describes how, from the perspective of Maharishi Vedic Science, the three-in-one dynamics of consciousness knowing itself (the Veda) generates "a rich spectrum of vibrational modes," which appear as all the forms and phenomena of the universe. Among these "resonant modes of consciousness," Dr. Hagelin points out, are the five fundamental categories of matter and energy—

the tanmatras—responsible for the material universe. He further explains that

> there is a striking correspondence between these five tanmatras and the five quantum-mechanical spin types of a unified quantum field theory: between the akasha or "space" tanmatra and the gravitational field; between the vayu or "air" tanmatra, which stands as a link between space and the other tanmatras, and the gravitino field; between the tejas or "fire" tanmatra, responsible for chemical transformations and the sense of sight, and the spin-1 force fields; and between the apas and prithivi ("water" and "earth") tanmatras and the spin-1/2 and spin-0 matter fields, respectively.

Dr. Hagelin's recognition of the identity of the five elements described in Maharishi Ayurveda and in modern physics, as well as many other correspondences, is an important step in the growth of understanding of this knowledge in the scientific community. The process of connecting different fields of scientific knowledge to their source in the unified field of natural law is creating a bridge between modern science and Maharishi Ayurveda that will allow scientists a more detailed and quantifiable understanding of how consciousness gives rise to matter.

The Three Doshas

According to Panchamahabhuta theory, the five elements combine to form three basic tendencies or operating principles of matter. These are known as the *doshas*. Dosha literally means "impurity." Doshas are considered impurities because as consciousness makes the transition from subjective to objective creation, it becomes "grosser" or more impure.

The three doshas are *Vata*, *Pitta*, and *Kapha*. Vata, according to Ayurvedic texts, is a combination of akasha and vayu; Pitta, of agni and jal; and Kapha, of jal and prithivi. In terms of the physiology, the three doshas represent three fundamental metabolic and psychophysiological principles underlying the functioning of the body, respectively: movement, metabolism, and structure.

The three doshas remind us of the three-in-one structure of pure consciousness, in which the three components—knower, process of knowing, and known—are called *Rishi*, *Devata*, and *Chhandas*. In fact, Vata, Pitta, and Kapha are the finest material expressions in the body respectively of Rishi, Devata, and Chhandas.

According to Maharishi Ayurveda each person has a different proportion of the doshas at birth. In many respects, this is like saying that we each have a different mixture of genes. Although all three doshas are present in everyone, most people have primarily a combination of two of the three, with one predominating. (For example, one might be classified as a Vata-Pitta, Vata-Kapha, or Pitta-Kapha nature.) Less common is the pure "mono-doshic" person, in which one dosha predominates. In rare instances, all three doshas may be equally in evidence.

Diet, age, weather, and countless other factors influence the proportion of doshas in the physiology. This has profound implications for health. When the doshas remain in their ideal proportion (which is different for different people), an individual remains healthy. When imbalance occurs—for example, if one of the doshas greatly increases or decreases in proportion to the others—the disease process begins. Susceptibility to different diseases, as well as the course of each disease, will vary depending upon which dosha predominates.

The goal of Maharishi Ayurveda is to recreate balance in Vata, Pitta, and Kapha. When the doshas are balanced, the inner intelligence of the body is reflected more completely at all levels of physiological functioning.

How can we know the ideal proportion of doshas in the physiology? How can we diagnose their current state of balance? The traditional texts of Ayurveda describe three means of diagnosis: sight, speech, and touch. The first two involve a physical examination and interview to determine the patient's medical history and current symptoms. The subtlest diagnostic technique, however, is pulse diagnosis, traditionally called *nadi vigyan*. The nadi, or pulse, contains information about the patient's entire physical and mental condition.

Pulse Diagnosis in Maharishi Ayurveda

One of the greatest experts in Maharishi Ayurveda was Dr. B. D. Triguna, past president of the All India Ayurveda Congress and member of the Indian government's Ayurveda research council. He was revered throughout his country and the world as a great *vaidya* (Ayurvedic physician), and a master of the subtle and sophisticated method of Ayurvedic pulse diagnosis. The president of India honored him with a special award for his long and distinguished career of devoted service to the health of the whole population. On numerous occasions, I have been both surprised and impressed with Dr. Triguna's remarkable ability to diagnose disease through the pulse alone. Again and again he diagnosed obscure conditions without any prior indication of the problem. On one occasion, a person was introduced and simply sat down. Dr. Triguna took his pulse and said, "This patient is colorblind." The man had indeed been colorblind since birth.

What does the physician detect in pulse diagnosis? It is certainly true that the pulse gives an overall indication of our heart and circulatory system. In Western medicine, one of the first diagnostic steps is to analyze the heart and circulatory system by measuring the pulse and taking the blood pressure. However, in Maharishi Ayurveda the diagnosis is far subtler and more comprehensive. When the physician puts his fingers on the radial pulse, he is not counting the number of pulses per minute as in Western medicine; he is determining the state of balance of the finer layers of the patient's physiology of matter.

The pulse in Maharishi Ayurveda is taken with three fingers: each finger is used to feel the state of one of the three doshas. The finger closest to the wrist determines the state of balance of Vata, the middle finger determines the state of Pitta, and the finger furthest from the wrist determines the state of Kapha. The physician also feels the quality of the pulse—its strength, regularity, and rhythm—with all three fingers. By analyzing the state of balance of each dosha, the physician can determine many things about the patient and his state of health.

From the viewpoint of Maharishi Ayurveda, the ideal of pulse diagnosis is when the vaidya feels the pulse, using the refined sense of touch, from the level of perfect balance and orderliness in his own highly developed awareness—from the level of his own self-interacting dynamics of consciousness. Starting from this level, his awareness precisely penetrates to the inner Self of the patient, fathoming the level where the infinite field of pure consciousness is becoming matter. From this level, he can thus feel the fluctuations of consciousness in the whole body.

Body Nature

One thing the physician determines is the patient's Ayurvedic body nature. We know that there are broad classifications of people—big, small, thin, muscular, fat, nervous, calm, etc.—yet modern medicine's knowledge of body or psychophysiological natures is very rudimentary. If we go back to the historical roots of Western medicine, however, we do find a long tradition of body typing. Hippocrates, the father of Western medicine, and Galen, the great Roman physician, classified the temperament of patients according to the proportion of four basic bodily fluids—blood, yellow bile, black bile, and phlegm—the so-called four fundamental humors. Variations of this and other approaches were used from the Middle Ages to the nineteenth century by many well known and respected physicians.

The first comprehensive and scientific approach to body typing in modern times was undertaken by W. H. Sheldon at Harvard University. In the 1930s and 1940s Dr. Sheldon surveyed a very large group of people and classified them into three main body types with many possible intermediate categories. These were named after the three main types of embryonic tissue from which all other tissues and organs eventually develop: the ectoderm, from which comes skin and nervous tissue; the mesoderm, from which muscle and connective tissue are derived; and the endoderm, from which most of our internal organs develop. Dr. Sheldon called the three basic types the ectomorph, the mesomorph, and endomorph. The ectomorph was in general tall and skinny, the mesomorph compact and muscular, and the endomorph fat and large. Dr. Sheldon also developed a very extensive scheme, involving many physical and psychological variables, for analyzing any individual according to the predominance or proportion of these three basic types. However, so far very little practical value has come from his research.

Other attempts at classification are generally based on exclusively psychological characteristics. For example, the idea that people could be classified as introverts or extroverts, or have high and low emotional reactivity, or,high and low stress reactivity (types A and B). Unfortunately none of the approaches has taken advantage of the extensive knowledge and practical experience of Maharishi Ayurveda.

The Ayurvedic system of health care contains extremely detailed knowledge of individual body natures. Actually, they are more accurately called "mind-body" natures, and by taking the pulse, the physician determines the natural psychophysiological makeup of an individual—the *prakriti*—which literally means "nature." An individual's prakriti represents the natural state of balance of the finer levels of the physiology of matter—the natural state of balance of the doshas (that is, the relative proportion of Vata, Pitta, and Kapha). Once the doctor knows the person's prakriti he can determine many factors. Most importantly he knows that each particular prakriti is susceptible to certain mental and physical disorders. The doctors can then, both from reading the pulse and also if necessary by physical examination, determine what is known as the *vikriti*.

The vikriti is the deviation of the doshas from their ideal state of balance. Further, each dosha has five subdivisions, or subdoshas, within it. A physician skilled in Maharishi Ayurveda can determine which doshas and subdoshas are imbalanced and thereby give a precise analysis of the patient's particular disorder. Determining the vikriti is of great value even if no serious disorders are present, because the physician can detect in the subtle imbalances in the pulse the seeds of future health problems long before they manifest. Once the diagnosis is made, the Ayurvedic physician prescribes therapeutic and preventive strategies. Many of these are highly individualized, based on the patient's prakriti and vikriti.

The Qualities of Vata, Pitta, and Kapha

To fully understand the body natures in Maharishi Ayurveda we must understand the qualities of each of the three doshas: Vata, Pitta, and Kapha.

The principle of Vata, as we have said, arises from akasha (space) and vayu (air). Vata is associated with movement within the body. It is involved with such vital functions as respiration, excretion, and neural control of sensory and motor function. People whose prakriti is predominantly Vata (or "Vata nature") are characteristically thin and light. They are rarely comfortable in the cold, dislike strong wind, and prefer warm, balmy weather, warm water, and warm food. They have a marked tendency toward dry skin, some constipation, and a variable appetite, sometimes strong, sometimes weak.

Vatas tend to be bright, quick to grasp new concepts, quick to learn, but poor on long-term memory. Vatas are also quick to conceive and initiate projects, but have difficulty in following through to the end. They are often highly creative, but they can be overemotional, with extreme mood swings. When Vatas feel good they can be euphoric.

When Vata dosha goes out of balance, there is a strong tendency toward worry and anxiety. People prone to this imbalance often overextend themselves even though they lack profound physical strength and stability. Vatas are susceptible to arthritis and hypertension. In general, they have a high sensitivity to all environmental stimuli, with a low threshold of pain. A classic Vata syndrome is well illustrated by the story of the princess and the pea. Even after 100 mattresses have been stacked on her bed, the princess is still disturbed by the presence of a tiny pea under the bottom mattress.

The second principal body nature, Pitta, is based on a predominance of Pitta dosha in one's prakriti, which is associated with heat and metabolism. The elements of agni (fire) and jal (water) are the basis of Pitta tendencies. Pitta is involved with such functions as digestion and thermoregulation. Pittas share some of the characteristics of the Vatas. They, too, tend to have agile minds; however, they have far more energy and staying power. They can be very aggressive, with a strong and penetrating intellect. They are well organized and can be good, authoritative decision-makers. Their bodies can take a lot of physical discipline and abuse, and they frequently take over-advantage of this attribute. General George Patton was almost certainly a characteristic Pitta nature. It is not pure coincidence that military people and athletes are frequently found to be Pitta natures.

When Pitta is imbalanced, Pittas will typically have trouble controlling their anger from time to time, if not frequently. They may be impatient and difficult to deal with. Pittas have strong digestion, but they must always have their food on time to maintain their equanimity. Peptic ulcer is the classic Pitta health problem. Whenever a skin disorder appears, regardless of the individual's body nature, it is an indication of a Pitta imbalance. Pitta-nature people have an aversion to hot weather and, regardless of weather, even the touch of their skin is noticeably warmer than that of a Vata person.

The third principal body nature, Kapha, is based on a predominance of Kapha dosha, which is associated with structure. In the fable of the tortoise and the hare, the tortoise is pure Kapha—slow and steady wins the race. Within the body, Kapha is concerned with the structural basis of the physiology. Its characteristics of solidity and inertia come from the elements of prithivi (earth) and jal (water). Structures such as membranes and connective tissue, which underlie the connectedness and stability of the body's different parts, are associated with Kapha.

Kaphas tend to be more heavily built, with somewhat oily skin, and often have dark and thick hair. Digestion tends to be slow, and Kapha people will often have a problem with overweight. Unlike Vatas, they are not easily disturbed, and unlike Pittas, they are slow to anger. Their minds are tranquil and steady, slow to learn but slow to forget. Because they are not easily upset, they often are warm, forgiving, and agreeable. Negative tendencies of excess or imbalanced Kapha can be dullness or sluggishness and the lack of creativity and ambition. Kaphas enjoy their heavy and deep sleep, but must have enough to be lively and focused the next day. The most predominant Kapha health disorders are asthma and obesity.

Research on Ayurvedic body typing has shown that the prakriti classification has a genetic basis. In one study researchers performed genome-wide SNP (single nucleotide polymorphism) analysis of 262 well-classified male individuals and found significant differences between prakriti natures. They also found a specific gene, PGM1, which correlates with Pitta. The functions of Pitta described in the ancient Ayurveda texts include digestion, metabolism and energy production. The PGM1 gene is in the center of many metabolic pathways including glycolysis, gluconeogenesis, pentose phosphate pathway, and galactose metabolism. The conclusion of the researchers was that the ancient system of Ayurveda has a valid basis in its analysis of individual dosha types.

A number of other studies have explored patterns of blood chemistry, genetic expression, physiological states, and chronic diseases associated with each dosha type. For example, one study found that triglycerides, total cholesterol, high LDL and low HDL concentrations—all common risk factors for cardiovascular disease—were reported to be higher in Kapha types compared to Pitta and Vata types. In a recent paper by Dr Fred Travis and myself we provide a review of the research and suggest specific experimental approaches to determine how different areas of the brain operate in each specific dosha type. We have further suggested using the termonology Brain/Body Nature in order to emphasize the importance of understand how basic differences in the wiring of the brain can account for dosha-specific mental and physical characteristics.

Further research should provide a fuller physiological understanding of the Ayurvedic psychophysiological typing system and thus help to introduce it more widely to the West. On the basis of this system, Maharishi Ayurveda provides a comprehensive nutritional and dietary program specifically designed for each nature. Further, it gives specific advice and procedures in regard to behavior, lifestyle, and physical fitness. Extensive knowledge exists in Maharishi Ayurveda concerning daily and seasonal biological rhythms with regard to individual body nature. On this basis certain daily and seasonal routines are prescribed for better health.

Let's consider why the knowledge of someone's body nature is valuable. Take the example of Anne, who was diagnosed as being angry. The modern physician, if he made the correct diagnosis, wouldn't really have much to offer such a patient. He probably would prescribe some mild sedative, or, if the condition worsened, a tranquillizer or painkiller. He might refer the patient to a psychologist or psychiatrist, who would probably prescribe more sophisticated medication.

Maharishi Ayurveda, on the other hand, would treat the patient very differently. In Maharishi Ayurveda, as in most systems of natural medicine, the orientation is toward the patient, not the disease. Who is my patient? What is his or her body nature? What are the tendencies toward imbalances that cause physical or mental disorders? After examining the patient, taking the pulse, and fully evaluating the patient's body nature, the physician would probably find, as in the case of Anne, that she was a Pitta. This would explain her tendency toward anger.

Further, the physician would question what foods the person had been eating. Certain foods are known to increase Pitta and can actually cause anger to be expressed more quickly. He would also examine other relevant aspects of the patient's life that might also aggravate Pitta and further note the time of day and season, since both these factors affect how the Pitta-nature person is behaving. Western-trained physicians who are also trained in Maharishi Ayurveda are inevitably impressed by the importance of understanding the patient's body nature before trying to prescribe a treatment or prevention program. To determine your own brain/body nature take the quiz at www.DharmaParenting.com.

Balance

Each body nature has its own strengths and weaknesses, and each person has his own genetic makeup and his own relative proportion of Vata, Pitta, and Kapha. Whatever that proportion is, it should be maintained in balance. According to Maharishi Ayurveda, disease occurs only when these three fundamental psychophysiological principles—Vata, Pitta, and Kapha—become aggravated or imbalanced.

Maharishi Ayurveda describes the various stages of imbalance that lead to disease. Perhaps most interesting, what we would consider in Western medicine to be a disorder's early symptoms are, in fact, the last stages in Maharishi Ayurveda. Through the knowledge of body natures and the three doshas, physicians are able to detect much earlier stages of disease.

For example, they may detect an imbalance caused by an excess of Pitta building up in some area of the body. There may be general symptoms of irritability or anger, but it is impossible at this stage to know how the imbalance will actually manifest. If the buildup becomes too great, then, according to Maharishi Ayurveda, some area of the body that is weaker and more prone to a Pitta imbalance will become the target for the excess Pitta. Instead of remaining a nonlocal mild state of weakness, the disturbance suddenly becomes localized and perhaps inflamed, causing the target organ or tissue to develop acute symptoms of a particular disease.

Since one site prone to Pitta imbalance is the stomach area, the patient might develop indigestion or even ulcers. These are just a few of the common signs of Pitta imbalance; it is important to note that symptoms can arise from imbalances in any of the doshas. The physician trained in Maharishi Ayurveda takes many different factors into account when diagnosing disorders and prescribing treatment for them.

In terms of modern medicine, we might understand this process of balance and imbalance in terms of one of the most important physiological principles—the principle of homeostasis. Homeostasis refers to the body's ability to maintain internal balance and stability even when there are changes in the environment.

There are many such mechanisms to keep all parts of our body in balance. Thus, the importance of balance is well understood in modern medicine. If one of these regulatory mechanisms is disturbed or overtaxed, for example in states of physical and mental stress, then the whole system suffers. Maharishi Ayurveda has very refined procedures for detecting these physiological imbalances and treating them before they actually manifest into a particular disease; this is one aspect of its successful prevention-oriented approach to health care.

Body Nature and Exercise

One of the most visible signs of the growing trend toward self-improvement in health is the fitness craze. Particularly in the United States more and more people have been taking up jogging, aerobics, or body building, or are involved in some type of diet or physical fitness program. There is a steady stream not only of diet, but also of exercise and fitness books. One can't help but see this as a healthy sign. People are at least waking up and remembering what it's like to get outside, breathe fresh air, and get the body moving again. The only trouble is that like many other things we do in America, we overdo. What started out as a positive direction of improving health has turned in many cases into a compulsive and overtaxing burden on our bodies.

Maharishi Ayurveda emphasizes the need to structure any exercise program according to age and body nature. Up to the age of 25, moderate to vigorous exercise on a regular basis is prescribed for all body natures. Over the age of 25, Ayurveda generally advises more moderate exercise for all natures, with the following specific recommendations for each nature.

Kaphas are the best suited for vigorous exercise, and it is essential that they exercise regularly. Otherwise, they will gain weight and tend to become lethargic. Pittas are often strong, muscular, and well-suited for exercise. For them moderate exercise is prescribed on a regular basis. Pitta people, like Type A individuals, have a tendency to overdo it. When exercising, they should not allow their competitive and sometimes driven spirit to push their physiologies too far, well beyond their normal capacities. This holds especially true for team sports. The Vata nature is more suited for very moderate exercise maintained on a regular basis. The Vata nature, in particular, needs to be careful about engaging in a fitness program that might be too strenuous. For Vata natures some of these programs could be detrimental rather than beneficial, causing exhaustion and imbalance.

Walking is one exercise recommended for all body natures. Other specific exercises are also recommended for all body natures. The most well-known of these are the Yoga asanas, a series of easy postures that stimulate the body in a systematic and natural way. Specific asanas can be recommended by Maharishi Ayurveda physicians to enhance the treatment of particular disorders.

The goal of all exercise in Maharishi Ayurveda is to rejuvenate the body and create bliss. Exercise should not be a strain to the physiology. The saying "no pain, no gain" is replaced by "gain without pain." For athletes, Maharishi Ayurveda prescribes effective training programs for optimizing performance without causing the physical discomfort and negative side effects characteristic of so many other programs. The body has full, unlimited potential. It is the stress and fatigue of exertion that inhibit the athlete from reaching fall athletic potential. When you remove the strain and fatigue, you remove the inhibiting factors. Once the stress and impurities are gone, then the athlete can perform at peak level. In fact, with Ayurvedic exercise, the potential for performance is unlimited. For both the average exercise buff and the professional athlete alike, Maharishi Ayurveda considers all aspects of the individual to create "a sound mind in a sound body."

Chapter 3

Digestion: The Key to Good Health

In Ayurveda, good digestion is the key to health. We generally think of digestion as the breakdown of food into smaller components that can be more easily absorbed and assimilated by the body. What we don't realize is that scientists have found that the digestive tract has a profound impact on many aspects of mental and physical health.

One interesting finding is within the digestive system is a second system called the enteric nervous system, which also help regulate digestion. This system is sometimes referred to as a "second brain," consisting of some one hundred million neurons—only one thousandth of the number of neurons in the brain, but still a very large number. It is embedded in the lining of our gut, all the way from the throat down. It makes use of more than 30 natural chemicals that are also found in the brain.

One of the most important is these is a neurotransmitter called serotonin, which plays a significant role in regulating mood. About 90% of all the serotonin in the body is located in the gut, and about 50% of the body's dopamine, a powerful reward chemical that controls both pleasure and addiction, is also located here. This "second brain" in our gut monitors the progress of digestion, keeps tract of nutrients, and evaluates the chemical nature (for example, the acidic or alkaline properties) of all the elements in the digestive tract.

Another fascinating area of research that links the ancient findings of Ayurveda with modern science has to do with the importance of the bacteria in our digestive system. It turns out that the types of bacteria in our gut can have marked effects on our immune system and even our brain. The community of microorganisms in the gut is called the microbiome and consists of about 100 trillion microbial cells. We have 10 times the number of microorganisms in our gut than we have cells in our body. The microbiome sends signals directly to the brain through the nervous system, and affects our immune functioning, which, in turn, is found to affect the development of our brain.

Recent research suggests that the human microbiome may have a role in auto-immune diseases like diabetes, rheumatoid arthritis, muscular dystrophy, multiple sclerosis, fibromyalgia, and perhaps some cancers. The development of certain critical immune cells seem to depend on the presence of certain bacteria in the microbiome. In addition, research shows that an imbalance of the microbes within the gut maybe also affect conditions such as anxiety, depression, and autism.

Our entire thinking has changed. These symbiotic microbes and their combinations may be the key to good health. What factors determines the type of bacteria we have in our gut? A significant one is our diet.

Individual Dietary Needs: Food is Medicine

In Maharishi Ayurveda, food is regarded as medicine. It would be unheard of for an Ayurvedic physician to prescribe a treatment for a particular disorder without taking into consideration first, the individual's body nature, and second, the particular foods that would be beneficial in correcting the physiological imbalance and preventing new ones from arising.

This is in great contrast to our current tradition of nutrition, which emphasizes an ideal or "best" diet for everyone. Of course, this best diet is constantly changing. Every few months, new best-selling diet books are prominently displayed across the country. Does anyone ever wonder why more and more books keep appearing? It must be for one of two reasons. Either there is a steady stream of brilliant Nobel prize-level scientific research being done in this area, or none of these new diet plans really works, so people keep trying new and "better" ones.

Most of the modern medical profession would agree with the latter. Quick and easy diet plans can sometimes produce some initial results, but in the long run the best approach seems to be a slow and steady process tailored to each individual and based on factors such as lifestyle and exercise.

If everyone is not already confused enough about new diet plans, what about the health food vitamin books? This is an area of huge controversy, not only between the medical profession and health food experts, but even among all the different health food experts themselves.

Diet and nutrition probably have more self-styled "experts" than any other health-related area. Who can you believe? Will vitamin C cure my cold? Will selenium protect us against cancer? These are some of the many issues that no one seems able to agree upon.

The health food people say the medical profession is too conservative and wants to control everything; therefore, it doesn't let the public in on the latest scientific findings. The medical profession is equally critical of the health food people, saying that based on only a few animal studies—or even without any research whatsoever—extraordinary and unsubstantiated claims are made for various vitamins, minerals, etc. The problem is that in both cases the conclusions about diet are based on incomplete knowledge, or knowledge that is constantly changing.

For example, the American Heart Association had mistakingly urged every person to reduce or give up saturated fats in milk, cheese, butter, and meat in favor of polyunsaturated fats. "Polyunsaturated" has become the byword for selling margarine and cooking oil for years. However, we now know that excess polyunsaturated fats may cause an increase in free radical reactions. This is a type of chemical reaction that may be at the basis of many disorders, including cancer and aging. More and more doctors are now recommending that a balance of fats be included in the diet, with monosaturated fats at the top of the list and polyunsaturated fats at the bottom. Yet many Americans still routinely buy polyunsaturated oils thinking that they are protecting their health.

Maharishi Ayurveda:
A Time-Tested Tradition of Nutrition

Maharishi Ayurveda, as we have said, places great emphasis on diet. Many foods and spices are considered to have a critical value for health, and therefore are recommended along with other treatment modalities. The most important difference between Maharishi Ayurveda and modern nutrition is Maharishi Ayurveda's concern for individual differences. If we were to analyze the various Maharishi Ayurveda diets, we would find that virtually all them conform to what modern nutritionists consider a balanced diet. They contain the right proportion and quality of fats, protein, minerals, vitamins, and carbohydrates. However, Maharishi Ayurveda very clearly states that no one diet is right for all people.

What is considered nourishing for one individual can actually be detrimental to another. For example, some sweets are said to be good for the Vata nature, while for a Kapha nature they may cause respiratory congestion or excess fat.

Hot, spicy foods are very good for Kaphas, yet they aggravate the digestion of a Pitta nature, leading to indigestion and a marked tendency toward anger. Each individual nature has its own needs.

Spontaneously, most of us have noticed over the years that certain types of food seem to be bad for us or are less appealing. On the other hand, sometimes we eat them anyway even though we know they have bad effects on us. This could be because of emotional imbalance, habit, ignorance, or failure to listen to the messages our physiology gives us. Maharishi Ayurveda provides a reliable, systematic body of knowledge that explains why we should or should not have certain types of food.

Maharishi Ayurveda is based on a long tradition of practical experience and a profound theoretical basis. But because of our often superior attitude toward "folk medicines," the dietary principles of traditional medical systems have unfortunately never been scientifically studied.

According to Maharishi Ayurveda, an important consideration when determining our diet is the strength of our digestion. Each body nature has a different strength of digestion, which is also influenced by factors such as climate and one's age and state of health. Most importantly, digestive strength depends upon the activity of our *agnis*. The agnis are the "fires of digestion," perhaps equivalent to our modern understanding of digestive enzymes. Weak agnis and improperly digested food can be a source of imbalance in the doshas. The by-product of undigested food is a substance which Ayurveda calls *ama*. The accumulation of ama aggravates the doshas and leads to all types of disorders.

The concept of disease caused by undigested food products is particularly interesting in the light of the recent research on our microbiome. Improper digestion and the accumulaltion of ama could aggravate our microbiome and cause problems throughout the body, such as a disturbance of the proper functioning of our immune system. Ayurveda speaks of a substance called *ojas*, which is the finest product of digestion. If the digestion is not effective then this can interfere with the production of ojas and disturb the formation of all the basic tissues, or *dhatus*, in the body and result in disease.

More research is necessary to identify the biochemical nature of ama and ojas. What is remarkable, however, is that these ancient concepts can now begin to be understood in modern scientific terms. Ayurveda many thousands of years ago understood the intimate connection between the digestive system and other key systems in the body, and precisely how the health of our body depends on the foods we eat.

Chapter 4

Biological Rhythms

A vital part of almost all traditional systems of medicine is knowledge of biological rhythms. Maharishi Ayurveda draws on a long-standing tradition that includes an especially rich and extensive knowledge of the impact of biological rhythms on diet, treatment of disease, behavior, and numerous other factors related to the individual body nature. In modern medicine we have only recently verified the importance of biological rhythms and, as a result, the field of chronobiology—the study of biological rhythms—has received widespread attention.

The most obvious biological rhythm is the diurnal or circadian rhythm, which results from the rotation of the earth on its axis every 24 hours. Many of our vital physiological signs, such as internal body temperature, as well as many biochemical and hormone levels, follow a daily pattern. Within our brain is an internal clock that helps keep track of time and set rhythms. Scientists have found a number of chronobiotic agents that can affect our daily rhythms. The most obvious of these are the environmental patterns of periods of light and dark that constantly reset our internal clock to match our environment. Also important are the foods we eat, the drugs and stimulants (such as coffee) we take, and the times we eat, rest, and exercise.

Anyone who has ever travelled knows that the biological resetting process, commonly referred to as "jet lag," can be very tiring and taxing. In the same way, we are all too aware of what happens if we stay up too late one night or miss meals. We put a strain on the body's own natural rhythms and, as a result, we create a temporary imbalance in the physiology, which must be corrected later on. Health, memory, emotions, job performance, and motor coordination have all been shown to be affected by shifts in our daily rhythms.

Perhaps the most important findings have been those related to modern medical treatment. Studies have shown that some drugs work differently at different times of the day. Dr. Franz Halberg, a pioneer in chronobiology, was one of the first scientists to document the importance of timing when treating cancer with radiation or with drugs.

Dr. Halberg found that a dose of radiation that killed mice at one time of day was much less toxic at another time. The tumor cells themselves were more sensitive to radiation at different times of the day. In the late 1960s he and his colleagues showed dramatic improvements in treating mouth tumors by properly timing the radiation treatment.

Since these early studies, numerous other studies have shown that the timing of both radiation and chemotherapy can make a marked difference in the effectiveness of the treatment. Drugs work at so many different levels of the physiology of matter, and each level has its own biological rhythm. DNA synthesis has its own rhythm, as do all the hormones, biochemicals, and even the cardiovascular system. For example, heart attacks strike three times more often at 9 A.M. than at 11 P.M.

The importance of understanding the body's biorhythms applies not only to the treatment of disease but also to its diagnosis. For example, there are numerous fluctuations in blood pressure as a result of the body's biological rhythms. Yet in a doctor's office, usually only one measurement at one time of the day is made to determine whether a patient has high blood pressure. It is easy to understand why misdiagnosis may occur. Some researchers have measured fluctuations in blood pressure and have used this information in diagnosis. For example, researchers have found that the pattern of these fluctuations in newborns can be used to predict their chances of developing high blood pressure when they grow older.

Maharishi Ayurveda takes into account varying biological rhythms in all phases of diagnosis, prevention, and treatment. It also takes into account the interaction of body nature and diet with these rhythms. The principal goal of Maharishi Ayurveda is to establish balance. Thus it places a special significance on establishing harmony between our individual rhythms and those of nature through various daily and seasonal routines. When we get out of the city into the countryside, we immediately notice the impact of nature's regularity. All the birds and animals wake up at a regular time; nature functions in a systematic and routine way. It should come as no surprise, then, that we are also designed to follow nature's rhythms. Maharishi Ayurveda therefore utilizes various therapeutic programs that reset our biological clocks to be in tune with those of nature.

The Effects of Seasonal Cycles on Our Health

One consideration in Maharishi Ayurveda quite new to Western understanding is the interaction of season, diet, and disease. While our current scientific understanding of seasonal changes is far from complete, recent research, especially on the pineal gland, has shown that animals are very sensitive to seasonal changes. As the day becomes longer, the amount of light stimulation increases. This has an effect on the secretion of melatonin, which in turn regulates other key glands, especially those involved in reproduction.

Modern medicine has uncovered some of the ways these seasonal changes might influence our health. For example, in 1984 Dr. Norman E. Rosenthal and colleagues at the National Institute of Mental Health identified a condition known as seasonal affective disorder (SAD), which results in depression. It occurs especially in northern countries and is caused by lack of sunlight, which influences the activity of the pineal gland.

According to Maharishi Ayurveda, seasonal changes can increase susceptibility to a number of disorders. The type of disorder can depend on the season and our body nature. The seasons themselves are related to the different doshas.

For example, at the beginning of Kapha season (early spring), the weather is often cold and damp and therefore more likely to cause an increase in Kapha. Especially in Kapha-nature people, this can create an imbalance resulting in colds, bronchitis, etc. On the other hand, at the beginning of Pitta season (early summer) Pittas, who are generally "hot" to begin with, may become imbalanced, leading to increased digestive problems and bouts of anger. Vatas are most susceptible to disease in Vata season, the cold and windy winter months. To protect the individual during these times of greater susceptibility, Maharishi Ayurveda makes many dietary and behavioral recommendations for each body nature.

The Vedic seers knew that the rhythms of the human body were tied to the rhythms of nature. They knew that for each person there was an ideal daily and seasonal routine to ensure that his or her rhythms were continually reset and resynchronized with those of the earth, moon, and sun. Further, they knew that the timing of a medical treatment was critical to its success. Therefore, all Maharishi Ayurveda treatments are individualized not only for the body nature, but for the time of day, the season, and the age of the patient.

Maharishi Ayurveda emphasizes that ideal health can only exist on the basis of an ideal relationship between human life and the laws of nature. The knowledge of the fundamental structures of the physiology of matter and of the physiology of consciousness—and of their underlying unity within the state of pure consciousness—provides a clear framework with which we can understand the technologies of the Vedic paradigm. This knowledge points to the reality that we, at a most fundamental level, are intimately connected with nature. It shows us that in the very process of realigning ourselves with the laws of nature, we can transform our personal experience and the world around us; we can transform our very physiologies. Maharishi uses a simple analogy to describe this relationship:

> It should be firmly established in the mind of every individual that he is part of the whole life of the universe and that his relationship to universal life is that of one cell to the whole body...The boundaries of the individual life are not restricted to the boundaries of the body, nor even to those of one's family or one's home. They extend far beyond those spheres to the limitless horizon of unbounded cosmic life.

Chapter 5

Medicinal Herbal Preparations

On a visit several years ago to the Philippines, I met with one of the top pharmacologists at the University of the Philippines in Manila. She was in charge of a large government project to scientifically evaluate and develop practical procedures for the use of herbal medicines. Quite a large percentage of the rural Filipino population uses herbal medicines, primarily because people cannot afford modern medicines and fear their potential side effects.

In many developing countries the cost of modern medicines is exorbitantly high. For example, I was told that many pharmacies in Brazil act like loan sharks, selling medicine on loan and charging very high interest rates. Another problem is that some powerful drugs we would never consider giving out without a prescription are readily available to people who may not be able to read the instructions. The pharmacologist in Manila had embarked upon a project to systematically evaluate the most commonly used herbs. It was a very well thought-out program, evaluating not only the pharmacological and clinical properties of each herb, but also the best method for the herb's growth, harvest, and conversion into medicine.

She explained that in each case they went into great detail in evaluating the herbs and their preparations. For example, an herbal text stated that for one particular medicine, only the top five leaves of a plant should be picked, and only during a particular time and season. The scientists attempted to find out why these instructions were given. As it turned out, when they had isolated what they thought was the most active ingredient, it was found to be most concentrated in the top leaves of the plant, and most abundant at the specified time and season.

Again and again they found that the ancient accounts held important secrets, which—to our loss—have been dismissed as hocus-pocus by the average scientist. But this woman was a very good and dedicated scientist, and as a result she was able to take advantage of extremely valuable traditional knowledge. The project was financed primarily by her government, with the long-term goal of reducing both health care costs and the dependence on Western medicine.

This type of project is by no means unique. Many countries have embarked on similar programs. In Kenya I talked with an eminent physiologist at the University of Nairobi who had a longstanding interest in Africa's systems of natural medicine. He pointed out that most of the experts lived in remote areas, and the so-called experts in the cities were often not the true masters of the traditional knowledge at all.

One reason why native medical traditions are being lost is that the knowledge is often passed only from father to son. Unfortunately, many of the younger generation are no longer interested in the old ways; they prefer to move to the cities, drawn by more material Western comforts. As a consequence, the older experts, rather than pass the knowledge of herbal preparations along to just anyone, allow it to die with them. This situation has clearly occurred in many cultures.

Compounding it is the loss of cultural integrity caused by conquest and foreign domination. We only have to look at the traditions of Native Americans to realize how easy it is for generations of knowledge to disappear in relatively few years.

Medicinal Herbs in Maharishi Ayurveda

One of the great contributions of Maharishi Ayurveda is its extensive knowledge of medicinal plants. We are extremely fortunate that Maharishi gathered the greatest Ayurvedic experts in this area to bring to light once again the knowledge of how these herbs work.

In Maharishi Ayurveda, the principle of complementarity holds that the physiologies of plants and animals are upheld by the same patterns of intelligence. Specifically, the sequence of biological information as stored in plants and minerals corresponds to the sequence of biological information in the human physiology. Herbal preparations function, Maharishi explains, like special biological "software" that supplies the essential program to re-establish the order and balance in the source code of the system.

To use another of Maharishi's analogies, the herbal preparations of Maharishi Ayurveda act like a set of tuning forks. Just as striking one tuning fork sets an identical one in sympathetic vibration, these herbs resonate in particular frequencies to restore the frequencies of self interaction associated with proper functioning in the various cells and tissues in the body. To say this a different way, the sequential unfoldment of intelligence in the herbal preparation resonates with the unfoldment of intelligence in the physiology of matter. It resets the correct sequence of unfoldment, removing any distortions that cause obstructions to the flow of intelligence. When these obstructions are removed, the body automatically corrects any imbalances that might lead to disease.

Maharishi Ayurveda contains the knowledge of how to use just the right preparations and combinations of very specific plants and minerals to treat a wide variety of disorders. Of particular interest are a group of herbal and mineral preparations known as rasayanas. Rasayanas, like the other herbal preparations in Maharishi Ayurveda, use this principle of complementarity. However, the function of rasayanas is both preventive as well as curative.

Some of the first studies on rasayanas were conducted at the Massachusetts Institute of Technology and involved a special preparation known as Maharishi Ayurveda Bhasma

Rasayana. This rasayana was developed by Dr. V. M. Dwive-di, an Ayurvedic physician for over 60 years, who had con-ducted research for some 30 years and had served on the graduate faculty of India's leading Ayurvedic university. He had worked closely with Maharishi for more than 10 years, and was one of the few remaining individuals in this gen-eration familiar with the highly complex and intricate pro-cess of preparing certain longevity promoting rasayanas. Dr. Tony Nader studied the effects of Dr. Dwivedi's specially prepared rasayanas and found strikingly beneficial effects. They were followed by a wide range of studies, particularly on the most important of the rasayanas, known as Maharishi Amrit Kalash.

Maharishi Amrit Kalash

Maharishi worked with other great Ayurvedic experts on herbal preparations. One was Dr. Balraj Maharshi, an advi-sor on Ayurveda to the government of India and perhaps the world's leading expert in *Dravyaguna*, the identification and utilization of medicinal plants. He had an extraordinary knowledge of over six thousand plants, many of which are very obscure and located in remote regions of India.

His great experience was illustrated a number of years ago at a conference in Brazil, which was attended by experts in natural medicine from Chile, Colombia, Bolivia, and oth-er South American countries. Also present was the head of a Brazilian botanical institute located near the Amazon, who had brought with her specimens of many different indigenous plants.

At one point the experts began to examine the plants and exchange knowledge about their medicinal uses. What was striking in this exchange was the very rich and complete knowledge Dr. Balraj brought out. Even though the plants were from an entirely different continent, he was able to bring out several more uses for, and details about, many more plants than were known by experts from the plants' country of origin.

Dr. Balraj's also helped in the formulation of Maharishi Amrit Kalash. Said to be the "king of rasayanas," Maharishi Amrit Kalash is intended to create balance from this level and establish the basis for fully integrated functioning of mind, body, behavior, and environment. Designed to be taken by all body natures, it is probably the only natural food supplement specifically formulated to develop higher states of consciousness.

Maharishi Amrit Kalash comes to us from the long history of the Vedic tradition; its fascinating story parallels the unfoldment of all the areas of Vedic knowledge through the self-interacting dynamics of consciousness. The Vedic literature records that at the dawn of creation, all the forces of nature assembled together to churn the primordial ocean of consciousness. This churning produced a few drops of ambrosia, known as amrit (the Sanskrit word for immortality), which was collected in a golden vessel called a kalash. This original preparation—the first rasayana—was used to restore the connection between immortal pure consciousness and the physiology to achieve perfection in life.

The formula for Maharishi Amrit Kalash—a compound of precious herbs from the thick forests and Himalayan mountainsides of India—was developed by sages under the leadership of Bhoja Raj, one of the revered kings of India, who distributed it to all his subjects so that they could develop perfect health. As with the entire range of Vedic wisdom, over the course of time the formula and its use became lost to the wider population; but it was closely guarded and handed down by a small number of Ayurvedic physicians in each generation. In modern times, the formula was given to Dr. Balraj.

Dr. Balraj knew that this rasayana was meant to be used on a mass scale for the benefit of society as a whole. He therefore waited for an opportunity to bring it to the world—which came when he met Maharishi Mahesh Yogi. In 1985, Maharishi asked Dr. Balraj, Dr. Dwivedi, and Dr. Triguna a question similar to one Bhoja Raj had posed to his advisors long ago: What could be done to eliminate disease and suffering and improve the quality of life of everyone in the world? Together with other eminent vaidyas, these three—the world's greatest exponents of Maharishi Ayurveda—restored the formula of Amrit Kalash in its completeness so that it could once again be widely available to promote perfect health in the whole population.

Maharishi Amrit Kalash is actually two different compounds composed of 23 herbs: "nectar" (M-4), and "ambrosia" (M-5). These compounds have been the subject of extensive scientific research in different parts of the world, at institutions including the National Institutes of Health and the National Cancer Institute, the Niwa Institute of Immunology in Japan, The Ohio State University College of Medicine, Loyola University Medical School, University of Kansas Medical Center, South Dakota State University, the University of Colorado, Indiana University, SRI International, and the University of California at Irvine.

These studies have shown the rasayana to have many potential benefits for health and longevity. Maharishi Amrit Kalash has been found to:

- inhibit tumor growth (in medical terminology, Maharishi Amrit Kalash is called anticarcinogenic— meaning that it both prevented the start (genesis) of cancer and decreased the size of existing tumors (this property is also referred to as antineoplastic),

- "scavenge" free radicals (it displayed antioxidant properties),

- have a positive influence on known cardiovascular risk factors, enhance the functioning of immune cells, and

- promote longevity and have anti-aging effects, and affect cell receptors in the brain and body.

In addition, Maharishi Amrit Kalash has been shown to be non-toxic and preventive.

The FDA and Herbal Preparations

If these herbal preparations have such good effects on health, why haven't they been used before in the West? The most important reason is that the traditional knowledge of herbs was lost—even in India.

Another very important factor is the U.S. Food and Drug Administration (FDA). In the United States, FDA regulations require an enormous amount of scientific investigation to be completed before any new drug or preparation can be prescribed for a specific disorder.

The caution with modern drugs is well-founded. We only have to remember the disastrous results with the premature use of drugs such as thalidomide, which caused widespread fetal abnormalities, to welcome the FDA's many regulations. To complete the necessary steps for testing a new drug, a pharmaceutical company must spend, over a five- to twelve-year period, hundreds of million of dollars.

Why does it cost so much? A battery of tests with different species of animals, ranging from rats to primates, must be done. Long-term clinical trials in humans must demonstrate not only that the drug has specific effects for a specific disease, but more importantly that its side effects are thoroughly known.

It is unfortunate, however, that in the United States the same regulations also apply to herbal medicine. There is a "grandfather" clause that allows preparations used for a long time in this country with no serious side effects to bypass all the regulations. Thus certain herbal tonics and the entire system of homeopathic medicine received a waiver under these regulations. However, this clause does not apply to herbal preparations used for thousands of years in other countries, such as China and India.

Although these preparations produce many verifiable health benefits without side effects, they are not permissible as prescription drugs. Therefore, getting an herbal medicine officially approved to treat a specific disease requires spending enormous sums of money.

Many commonly used drugs have been derived from plants. For example, the active ingredient in aspirin is a synthetic derivative of a compound present in the bark of the willow tree. One of the most powerful drugs used in treating heart attacks, digitalis, was derived from the flowering plant foxglove, and the chemotherapeutic agent vincristine comes from the Madagascar periwinkle.

Unfortunately, only a fraction of the knowledge of medicinal plants has ever been utilized. In fact, at a lecture I gave in Egypt some years ago to a conference of physicians, it was pointed out that what had survived from the great systems of herbal medicine were mostly not the useful ingredients, but rather the potentially harmful ones—such as opium, cocaine, caffeine, and nicotine—considered by most pharmacologists as poisons.

Another serious roadblock to their acceptance is that most preparations of herbal medicine involve whole plants or many plants, as well as minerals. Drug companies are generally reluctant to develop and patent such complex preparations. Their primary approach is to isolate and then patent an active ingredient or some similar synthetic product, thus ensuring the protection of their multi-million dollar investment. While financially logical, this approach contains a great medical fallacy.

Even in simple herbal preparations there is usually more than one active chemical ingredient. Although one chemical may be the most important for producing the medicinal effect, the other ingredients often serve to counteract any possible side effects. This is the principle of synergy in Maharishi Ayurveda. In contrast, most modern drugs contain only one active ingredient. It almost always produces side effects. Thus the whole plant or herbal preparation is more holistic and safer than a modern drug. When we isolate the active ingredient, we take some partial knowledge from the plant but lose its holistic wisdom.

Many herbs, tonics, various kinds of Chinese medicine, and similar products abound in certain kinds of health food stores. Proponents sometimes make what the FDA considers to be illegal and often untrue claims. I have spoken directly with several top FDA officials who said quite frankly that they just don't have the personnel to enforce all of the agency's regulations. Some countries, such as Switzerland, have altered their laws so medical officials can grant licenses to produce and sell beneficial herbal compounds as drugs with specific claims.

The whole picture becomes really complicated when we realize that in many systems of traditional medicine, certain common foods are considered drugs because they can help cure very specific conditions. Should the FDA regulate honey or milk since they are said in the traditional system of Indian medicine to be good for curing certain diseases? Hardly. But there must eventually be a change in our FDA laws, and it probably will have to be initiated from the top.

When former President Nixon first visited China, he became very interested in Chinese medicine, specifically in acupuncture. A directive came from the president's office to the National Institutes of Health to look into Traditional Chinese Medicine or TCM, and suddenly a lot of money was available for research in this area. While TCM is still a long way from receiving blanket approval, certain procedures such as acupuncture are officially practiced in many states as long as the technician is licensed by an approved agency.

I have visited China several times. I have spoken with scientists, given lectures at universities and at the Colleges of TCM, and taken part in a lively private meeting with the Minister of Health. TCM includes meditation, acupuncture, herbal medicines, holistic diets, breathing techniques, longevity treatments, and an enormous variety of exercise, including the martial arts. Traditional medicine is part of the essential fabric of life in China.

In the early morning many hundreds of people, including the very elderly, can be seen exercising in parks, squares, and on rooftops. Herbal medicines are everywhere; one especially finds preparations formulated to promote the extension of life. From early childhood on, the Chinese know that a certain food will produce a hot or cold effect on the body, and that disease is caused by an imbalance in the underlying forces of yin and yang. When people go to the hospital, they now have a choice of Western or traditional Chinese medical treatment.

In 2015 the Nobel Prize in medicine was given to Youyou Tu for her study of the effects of the TCM herb artemisia annua as a cure for the treatment of malaria. This award is a great achievement for both traditional medicine and integrative medicine, since it brings recognition of the great knowledge contained in these ancient traditions.

A number of international organizations, such as the World Health Organization, encourage the revival of traditional systems of medicine. One of the most useful programs that has been developed is the collection onto one large computer database of all research done on the different herbs. This database, known as Napralert, or Natural Products Alert, is located at the University of Illinois in Chicago and provides comprehensive information for developing countries.

Unfortunately, so much knowledge in many of these traditional systems of medicine has been lost over time, especially with the current emphasis on modern medicine. It is essential that there be a rapid revitalization of traditional systems of medicine in all countries. With its comprehensive approach, Maharishi Ayurveda can help restore each system of traditional medicine to its full potential.

For example, the extensive knowledge contained in Maharishi Ayurveda about plants and mineral preparations should be a great resource in rediscovering the uses of medicinal plants in each country. The materia medica of Ayurveda is very complete. Using it as a basis for comparison will ensure that the materia medica for all systems of traditional medicine become more complete and comprehensive.

Research on Common Spices and Herbs

Scientists at established universities have begun to conduct research and clinical trials on the numerous medicinal spices and herbs. We can see this clearly if we examine the current research on three common spices in Ayurveda and other systems: turmeric, ginger, and black cumin.

> **Turmeric.** Turmeric (Curcuma longa) is a common spice in both India and China. Marco Polo was said to have discovered it in 1280, and he believed it was related to the more expensive saffron spice because of its yellow color. We now realize that turmeric is far more than merely a common spice. It is a super-food that has numerous beneficial effects for health.

Research on turmeric and especially curcumin (diferuloylmethane), its active ingredient, is more extensive than almost any other natural product. It has been estimated that turmeric and curcumin have been the subject of over 5000 peer-reviewed and published biomedical studies, and there are 600 potential preventive and therapeutic applications, as well as 175 distinct beneficial physiological effects. Most of the initial research on turmeric and curcumin has been done on animals and in the laboratory, but an increasing number of new studies are being done on humans. In September 2012, the U.S. National Institutes of Health had seventy-one registered clinical trials completed or underway to study curcumin for a variety of clinical disorders.

Ginger. Ginger (Zingiber officinale) is a member of a plant family that includes cardamom and turmeric. For thousands of years ginger has been used as both a spice and an herbal medicine. It was a highly sought commodity exported from India to the Roman Empire, and then controlled by Arab merchants for centuries. The popular "Gingerbread Man" cookie shape is said to be the inspiration of Queen Elizabeth I of England. PubMed lists over 1700 research papers on ginger, revealing important properties which include antimicrobial, antioxidant, anti-inflammatory, antiemetic, antidiabetic, and anticancer.

Black Cumin. Black Cumin (Nigella sativa) is a well known spice in the Middle East and India. Less familiar in the West, it is often confused with the more common cumin (Cuminum cyminum). Black cumin grows well in the Mediterranean region and in western Asian countries including India, Pakistan and Afghanistan. It has a long history and is described in many ancient texts, including the Bible. Black cumin seeds were found in the tomb of the Egyptian Pharaoh Tutankhamen, and Hippocrates commented on its many benefits. In our own time, the results of modern research have begun to support a famous statement attributed to the Prophet Mohammad, referring to it as "a remedy for every disease except death."

Over 500 studies have been conducted in the last two decades showing the extraordinary range of benefits conferred by black cumin and its components including: anticancer, antioxidant, antimicrobial, anthelmintic, antischistosomiasis, renal protective, gastroprotective antiulcer, anti-inflammatory, immunomodulatory, analgesic, antipyretic, hepatoprotective, antiasthmatic, bronchodilator, calcium antagonist, diuretic, antihypertensive, antiatherosclerotic and antihyperlipidemic, antihypoglycemic and antidiabetic effects.

The Future of Medicinal Plants

Plants are one of our least expensive and yet potentially most important resources for the improvement of health. One of the most serious problems today is the preservation of invaluable plant materials in every country that are on the verge of becoming extinct. Whole species of medicinal plants are being totally eliminated as forests and jungles are claimed for agricultural purposes. The medicinal plants of every country offer the potential for greatly reducing health care costs. If this resource is destroyed, it will be a loss not only to the people and economy of the country, but also to the world.

Maharishi Ayurveda is helping to educate scientists and health care professionals about the invaluable potential of medicinal plants. It is not an easy process, since we have come to depend almost completely upon synthetic drugs—even with their host of unwanted side effects.

The benefits of medicinal plants, however, are vast: drastic reductions of health care costs; elimination of many of the abhorrent side effects of modern drugs; the offer of new treatments, as well as new methods of prevention, for diseases considered incurable by modern medicine; and most of all the natural promotion of health and longevity.

Chapter 6

The Network of Intelligence

Maharishi Ayurveda offers many therapeutic techniques that are designed to enliven the body's own inner intelligence and create balance at the finest layers of the physiology of matter. The most fundamental of these programs are the consciousness-based techniques. We have already briefly mentioned the Transcendental Meditation technique and in the next chapter we will consider the Vedic Sound program. We have also described the use of pulse diagnosis and prescription of specific changes in lifestyle based on an understanding of the state of balance of the individual mind/body nature. In addition, Maharishi Ayurveda includes a wide vareity of programs designed to reach the inner network of intelligence through our senses.

One such therapy is Maharishi Gandharva Veda music. Vedic texts explain that the melodies of Gandharva Veda, the classical music of the ancient Vedic civilization, are "the melodies of nature"—the intelligence and rhythms of nature expressed in music—and therefore have significant therapeutic value.

Modern science has glimpsed this principle of sounds and melodies at the basis of physical and biological phenomena. In the early 1980s, while studying DNA and molecular evolution, Dr. Susumu Ohno made an interesting discovery. He found that the sequences of nucleotides in DNA that code for life formed patterns similar to those seen in music. Translating these sequences into sheet music, he found that they sounded like the classical music of the Baroque and Romantic periods. The musical patterns within cancer-causing oncogenes sounded somber and funereal, while those within genes that form the lens of the eye sounded airy and playful. While these studies are preliminary and require a degree of extrapolation, they suggest that certain universal patterns underlie human creativity as well as nature's creativity.

The timeless knowledge of Maharishi Ayurveda takes a more expanded view: there is order and periodicity in the universe, whether in the motion of the planets or in the genes. The patterns and rhythms of nature are expressions of the fundamental rhythms of the unified field of natural law.

The goal of Maharishi Gandharva Veda therapy, the application of music to health, is to help attune the body to the underlying harmony and orderliness of nature and thereby re-establish physiological balance. Similarly to Vedic Sound therapy, the sounds of Gandharva Veda, according to Maharishi Ayurveda, resonate with the body's finest layers of matter and re-enliven the junction point between these structures and the sequence of natural law at their basis in consciousness. The sounds are very soothing, pleasing, and enlivening.

Preliminary research has shown that subjects listening to this music demonstrate a marked reduction in breathing—in some cases with repeated periods of respiratory suspension. These respiratory suspensions were not followed by compensatory hyperventilation, but by low respiration rates. Subjective experiences, especially during these periods of respiratory suspensions, were described in terms of greater inner clarity, wakefulness, and bliss. As mentioned earlier, periods of respiratory suspension have been seen in subjects practicing the Transcendental Meditation technique and have also been correlated with subjective reports of the experience of unbounded consciousness.

Gandharva Veda therapy helps to create happiness and bliss, nourish the senses, and clear away imbalances. Gandharva Veda therapy also attunes us to the natural rhythms and cycles of nature. It divides the day into eight important three-hour time periods and prescribes specific types of music to attune us to the laws of nature in each of these periods. These periods are known to be governed by the different doshas; listening to the appropriate Gandharva Veda music at each time is meant to bring balance to the doshas in the physiology.

Aromatherapy

Another approach of Maharishi Ayurveda that uses the senses as a way of influencing the body's intelligence network is Aromatherapy. The patient is treated with certain aromas depending on which doshas or subdoshas are imbalanced. The aromas are usually in the form of oils that have been distilled or extracted from plant material. The purpose of the aroma is to calm or rebalance the doshas.

There is considerable research on the sense of smell in Western science. Unlike other senses, the sense of smell is not relayed to the brain via one of its central structures (the thalamus), but instead passes directly from the nose to an older part of the brain (the amygdala), which is closely connected to the regulation of emotional reactions. It is clear that certain aromas have the ability to evoke vivid emotional memories.

In terms of Maharishi Ayurveda, the purpose of the aroma is again to reset the correct sequential unfoldment of intelligence in the body. It has been proposed that different aromas introduce certain sensory information in the brain, stimulating specific electrophysiological and biochemical pathways that help to remove imbalances and enable the body's inner intelligence to again flow in an orderly and unobstructed manner.

Pranayama

One way to engage the body's intelligence network is through breath. As part of Maharishi Ayurveda, there are specific Vedic breathing exercises, called *pranayama*, which enhance the connection between mind and body and help re-establish balance in the doshas.

Breathing exercises are important therapeutic strategies in many traditional systems of medicine. Research suggests how breathing exercises might affect the brain and therefore the entire body. One study measured the influence of breathing exercises on brain waves. The results suggest that patterns of EEG dominance can be affected by the breath.

Measurements show that our breathing follows regular cycles. These nasal cycles involve the rhythmic switching of the airflow from the right to the left nostril over a period of about 90 minutes. When the airflow is predominantly through the right nostril, higher relative amplitudes of EEG activity are found in the left hemisphere, and vice versa.

Further, studies show that the balance of dominance can be shifted by intentionally altering the nasal cycle through pranayama. For example, closing the right nostril and gently breathing through the left nostril causes increased EEG activity in the brain's right hemisphere, and the opposite occurs when the breathing is switched. One study found that changes in EEG patterns occurred almost instantaneously, and after 10 or 15 seconds a long-lasting shift in EEG dominance occurred. These results suggest that by altering the nasal cycle through specific pranayama exercises, we can alter neurophysiological functioning in the brain.

Many years ago Nobel Laureate Dr. Roger Sperry and his collaborator, Dr. Michael Gazzaniga, found that patients who had undergone surgical separation of the right and left cerebral hemispheres of the brain to prevent the spreading of epileptic seizures showed unusual characteristics. These patients behaved as if each of the two sides of their brains had a mind of its own: the left side saw the world from a more analytical, scientific perspective, while the right side saw the world with a more synthetic, artistic vision. This research inspired other studies into the nature of the brain: over the years, researchers have tried to locate specific control centers in the brain's structure responsible for specific physiological functions. Although the strict division of the brain into right and left is now considered an oversimplification (many processes actually involve whole-brain activity), it has nevertheless proved to be extremely useful.

One of the goals of pranayama is to establish balance in the physiology and psychology. Perhaps by rhythmically altering the nasal cycles, we can establish better integration between the two hemispheres of the brain, between our so-called "scientific" and "artistic" modes of psychological functioning. Since the brain controls all physiological functions, it is reasonable to assume that breathing exercises might affect other parts of the body via the nervous system.

In Maharishi Ayurveda, these pranayama breathing exercises are used as a general prevention measure and are prescribed for specific conditions depending upon the particular dosha that is imbalanced.

Maharishi Panchakarma Therapy

Maharishi Panchakarma therapy involves purification procedures that are prescribed according to body nature. These procedures influence the body's intelligence network through a variety of means, including herbalized oil massages, herbal steam baths, herbal elimination treatments, special eye and nose treatments, and a variety of dietary and behavioral programs.

The Panchakarma procedures, according to Maharishi Ayurveda, restore balance within the system, specifically balance among the doshas. Ayurveda states that the body is permeated by hollow channels called *shrotas* that must be kept open to promote and maintain health. Panchakarma removes any obstruction in the shrotas and thus allows the body's inner intelligence to flow freely. Because of its strengthening and refreshing effects on the mind and body, it is also referred to as "rejuvenation therapy."

Studies show that Maharishi Panchakarma improves mental and physical health and reduces biological age. In one study researchers found that with Panchakarma, patients demonstrated improved mental health characterized by significant reductions in negative moods (including anxiety, depression, and fatigue) and increased vigor as compared with control subjects who were given knowledge about Maharishi Ayurveda but not the actual treatment. In a similar study, Panchakarma subjects showed significant improvements in energy, vitality, well-being, strength, stamina, appetite, digestion, and rejuvenation compared with controls.

Maharishi Panchakarma also affects cholesterol levels. A study completed at the University of Freiburg in Germany found a 10% decrease in cholesterol after one to two weeks of Maharishi Panchakarma treatment, compared with no change in a control group. There was also a decrease of 8.7% in LDL. These results have been replicated and extended by a recent study in the United States, which found an acute decrease in cholesterol immediately following Maharishi Panchakarma treatment and an increase in HDL levels three months later. In addition, lipid peroxide, a measure of free radical activity, was found to rise during Panchakarma treatment and then to decrease to lower levels three months later. (The temporary increase might be associated with the purifying nature of this treatment, with the consequent beneficial effect of purification being seen in the eventual lower levels.) Finally, a neuropeptide known as VIP has a number of actions, one of which is increased blood flow in the arteries supplying the heart; VIP was found to increase by 80% three months after treatment.

One other area of research concerns the use of sesame oil, the primary oil used in several treatments. In one of the

Panchakarma programs known as abhyanga, herbalized sesame oil is massaged over the entire body with a pressure and speed that depends upon the person's physical condition and body nature. Maharishi Ayurveda recommends that everyone do a daily sesame oil massage at home. Dr. D. Edwards Smith has been researching the effects of sesame oil. In one procedure known as gandush, which involves applying the oil inside the mouth, he found a significant reduction in oral bacterial counts.

Dr. Smith hypothesizes that linoleic acid, which comprises 40% of the fatty acids in sesame oil, may be metabolized into a natural antibacterial agent. Linoleic acid is present in the skin and is known to inhibit the growth of certain pathogenic bacteria. Linoleic acid has also been found to be an and-inflammatory agent. Dr. Smith and his co-worker Dr. John Salerno have published several research papers on the effects of linoleic acid and sesame oil as preventive chemotherapeutic agents against cancer. They have found that both linoleic acid and sesame oil selectively inhibit the growth of both colon and skin cancer cells in vitro (in a cell culture).

Chapter 7

The Mistake of the Intellect

In Maharishi Ayurveda, it is the intellect that inhibits us most from seeing our true inner nature, and it is the intellect that is ultimately responsible for our state of health. The intellect has the ability to shift our attention in one of two directions: either outward toward the diversity of life, or inward toward the unity of consciousness. Maharishi Ayurveda refers to a condition known as *pragyaparadha*, the "mistake of the intellect." In this condition, the intellect becomes so absorbed in the diversified value of creation that it cannot perceive the underlying unity of life. According to Maharishi Ayurveda, this is the basic cause of imbalance in the physiology.

To eliminate this mistake, we must reawaken within our awareness its underlying unified value. We must shift our attention to the wholeness of consciousness by using strategies that are able to realign every aspect of the physiology of matter with the most fundamental level of our physiology of consciousness.

Maharishi further explained that imbalances arise in the body, leading to pain, sickness, and suffering, whenever the process of manifestation of intelligence into matter loses its self-referral quality—that is, becomes disconnected from the underlying unity of life:

> Balance is a state of satisfaction. Deviation from balance is dissatisfaction. Pain and suffering result from imbalances. Anywhere in the process of manifestation of intelligence into matter or in the reaction of matter with matter, any-where in those space-time boundaries that the self-referral condition is unavailable, there is pain and suffering.

The intellect, Maharishi pointed out, plays the central role in maintaining balance, by maintaining its complete coordination with the Self. "If some abnormality develops in the intellect, then, even if something is right, one would comprehend it to be wrong. It is the fineness of the intellect which maintains the self-referral state. ... If the intellect is in a balanced state then everything is brilliant, clear, full of sat-isfaction, and blissful."

Through the mistake of the intellect, the diverse expres-sions of the self-referral intelligence in our physiology of consciousness "forget" their basis in the unmanifest, unified state of pure consciousness.

The unity value of pure consciousness is lost to our view; the doshas lose their connection to their source, and thus they become imbalanced. When imbalances arise in the physiology of consciousness, they in turn create (for example, through improper diet and poor daily routine) imbalances and disease in the physiology of matter.

The purpose of the approaches of Maharishi Ayurveda is to reset the sequential unfoldment of the expressions of natural law in our physiology of matter. They fulfill this purpose by helping us attune ourselves to the most fundamental level of our physiology of consciousness—pure consciousness, the state of perfect balance. This process of resetting automatically corrects the mistake of the intellect, since it enables us to wake up to our own inner Self.

This is how we can spontaneously and automatically restore perfect balance in the physiology. The inner intelligence of the body, the "memory" of the unified value of pure consciousness, is reawakened, and the body's own homeostatic mechanisms begin to function optimally, thus eliminating disease, restoring health, and promoting longevity. Maharishi explains how the purpose of Maharishi Ayurveda to promote longevity is fulfilled by maintaining "that state of togetherness of the fundamental values of life":

> Veda is immortal. Pure knowledge is immortal. The organizing power of nature inherent in the structure of pure knowledge is immortal. Thus balance is immortal, and if, through the knowledge of Ayurveda, one maintains balance in the physiology, mind, and behavior, then that is the direction of long life.

Vedic Sounds

According to Maharishi Ayurveda, it is Vedic sounds that structure and direct all matter and energy. They are the basic impulses of natural law that are responsible for all creation. Like seeds about to sprout, these impulses of nature's intelligence are not yet manifest, but are vibrating within themselves, forming the dynamic, self-referral fabric of the unified field. This unmanifest fabric of sound is the basis of our own physiology of consciousness.

Contained in seed form in these sounds is the blueprint of the manifest universe, in the same way that DNA contains in seed form the blueprint of the entire body. There is an intimate relationship between the unmanifest seed sounds in consciousness and their manifest expressions in matter. In the Vedic tradition this relationship is called *nama* (name) and *rupa* (form): the name is composed of different sounds— different frequencies of self-interaction; the form is the material expression that spontaneously arises from the sequential unfoldment of the sound or name. In other words, the form is simply a more manifest expression of the vibratory impulses in the name.

Again, we can see an analogous situation in DNA, where each gene within the DNA codes for a specific protein. The name is the information coded in the sequence of nucleotides on the DNA, and the form is the three-dimensional shape of the particular protein.

Vedic sounds are the basis of one of the approaches of Maharishi Ayurveda, which makes use of this intimate relationship between the seed sounds and their manifest forms in the body. The body, at its finest level, is just the expression of sound. As we just saw, disease and disorders arise due to pragyaparadha, when the material forms in the body become disconnected from their self-referral basis in pure consciousness. That is, the sequential unfoldment of sounds has been disrupted, has gotten out of its proper sequence.

The Vedic Sound approach of Maharishi Ayurveda is designed to reset the unfoldment of intelligence in our body to match its original perfect pattern in pure consciousness, and thus to remove any physiological imbalances. This principle of resetting the correct unfoldment of intelligence lies at the heart of the therapeutic strategies of Maharishi Ayurveda.

By way of analogy, consider an orchestra rehearsing Beethoven's Symphony No. 7. There is a perfect orderliness and beauty in the musical piece, which is represented on a gross manifest level by the notes on the musical score. The conductor, the "DNA" of the orchestra, has in his awareness exactly how the piece should unfold and how all the instruments should relate to each other; he is responsible for the orderly unfoldment of the intelligence in the music. At any stage of the piece, he can identify if a note is played out of sequence, or if a wrong note has been played. The conductor compares what is being played to the pattern of the unmanifest musical score that he holds in his awareness. If an error occurs, he stops the rehearsal and indicates where a correction must be made. In this activity, he is actually reconnecting the performance of the orchestra with the patterns of musical intelligence in his own awareness. He enlivens this intelligence in the awareness of the musicians; they spontaneously correct their performance, and the music proceeds. This process resets the perfect sequential unfoldment of the music.

In the physiology, we can see how this principle operates in the development of cancer: cancer cells are renegade cells that have declared mutiny on the body. The sequence of expression of knowledge in DNA (the name) has become distorted; as a result their material form also becomes distorted, as well as dangerous. The cells have lost their memory of what they are supposed to do, and instead of functioning as normal cells, they produce large quantities of growth factors and begin to divide and spread at an unchecked rate, exhausting the body's resources for their growth.

The use of Vedic sound is designed to reconnect the material structure of the physiology with the self-referral intelligence at its basis. This enlivenment of the inner intelligence of the body helps the body to spontaneously heal itself. In the case of cancer, the sequence of the expression of DNA would regain its normal pattern, and the cells would thus regain their memory of how to function as healthy cells.

Researchers at Ohio State University have found experimental evidence suggesting that the sounds of the Vedic literature have a beneficial effect on re-enlivening the inner intelligence of the body. The effects of Vedic sounds were compared to those of hard rock music, and no sound, on the growth of cells in culture. Five types of human cancer cells (lung, colon, brain, breast, and melanoma) and one normal cell type were tested in four experiments. The recordings of Vedic sounds and hard rock were adjusted so that the degree of loudness was similar for both. Vedic sounds decreased growth in all the cancer cell types. In the presence of hard rock music, cell growth was generally increased, although the effects were not consistent.

Maharishi Ayurveda prescribes specific Vedic sounds according to the specific physiological disorder. As the impulses of sound reverberate in the awareness, a kind of sympathetic resonance occurs; they act as a template that can restore the body to a state of balance.

Discovery of the the Veda in Human Physiology

Dr. Tony Nader, working closely with Maharishi, found that there is an exact, one-to-one correspondence between the various aspects of the Vedic literature and the anatomical structures which together comprise the human brain and nervous system. Thus the Veda is found not only within our consciousness, but throughout our physiology.

This remarkable finding is the subject of Dr. Nader's book, entitled *Human Physiology: Expression of Veda and the Vedic literature—Modern Science and Ancient Vedic Science Discover the Fabrics of Immortality in the Human Physiology.*

This discovery makes clear that all the creative qualities of consciousness (the Vedic literature), which are the basic unmanifest structure of pure consciousness, are also found in unmanifest form in the different structures of the human brain and nervous system, such as the cortex, hypothalamus, thalamus, etc. The internal mathematical structure of each branch of the Vedic literature precisely corresponds to the internal structure of each of these aspects of the anatomy. Thus, our own physiology is the Veda made manifest.

The Vedic Sound therapy of Maharishi Ayurveda is one practical application of this discovery. Its full implications are vast and far-reaching. Through the technologies of Maharishi Vedic Science and Maharishi Ayurveda, all the aspects of the Veda—all the aspects of natural law that govern the universe with infinite creativity and infinite organizing power, and without problems or mistakes—become fully awake not only in our consciousness, but throughout our physiology. Then our lives and our health will be supported by the total potential of natural law, free from mistakes and problems.

The Individual and the Environment

Maharishi Ayurveda uses several therapeutic strategies that take into account the relationship of the individual to the environment. For example, thre is Maharishi Sthapatya Veda, which focuses on your near environment, the health of your home and the building you work in. And still another is Maharishi Jyotish, which considers your far environment and provides a mathematical approach to diagnose and prognosticate disease.

Through Maharishi Jyotish the position of any event in the sequential unfolding of natural law can be precisely known; therefore its past, present, and future can be accurately described. A medical condition can thus be perceived with remarkable accuracy in context of its history and prognosis. All that is required is the knowledge of a few key elements.

This principle is a familiar one in Western physiology and medicine. For example, we know that the cells of a human embryo evolve in highly specific ways, due to the information encoded within the cells themselves. At any given stage, we can accurately predict the embryo's development and its reaction to any changes in its environment.

Likewise, through blood tests we can see indicators of potential, nascent, or existing disease. Given these indicators, we can successfully predict what will occur in the future. However, Maharishi Jyotish, instead of relying on gross, external measurements (such as blood samples) used by Western science, relies on precise, mathematically derived descriptions of nature's unfoldment.

In Maharishi Ayurveda, Jyotish is used for both prevention and cure. As prevention, it allows the physician to perceive and correct in advance potential imbalances in a patient. As cure, it enables the physician to neutralize negative environmental influences that may be hindering the effective action of other Ayurvedic therapies.

A second strategy, Maharishi Yagya, is the applied aspect of Jyotish. Yagyas are specific Vedic performances, which utilize Vedic sounds to reset the patterns of sequential unfoldment of nature's intelligence in the mind, body, and environment. We can think of these performances as preventive maintenance. Yagyas are said to prevent dangerous conditions before they arise within the physiology of matter by working on the level of the physiology of consciousness.

For individuals with high blood pressure, doctors often prescribe medication and a restricted diet. This is preventive medicine on the level of the physiology of matter. By having these people practice TM regularly, doctors are applying preventive medicine on the level of the physiology of consciousness. In this sense, Transcendental Meditation itself is also a type of yagya.

Because of their broad range of influence, yagyas can be used either as individual or collective health measures. The individual body is made up of a collection of cells; society is like the body in that it is made up of a collection of individuals. Yagyas can be used to help neutralize imbalance in society and thus produce good effects on the overall collective health and quality of life.

What is unique about yagyas is the level of precision and sophistication involved. They are equivalent to the most advanced type of engineering, such as that involved in a flight to the moon. The difference is that a yagya is engineering on the deepest level of natural law. This is Vedic engineering:

engineering on the level of pure consciousness. Those skilled in the application of yagyas are highly trained in the technologies of consciousness. They must be able to maintain that most silent and unified state of consciousness in their own awareness while they reset the unfoldment of nature's intelligence through these Vedic performances.

In summary, all the approaches of Maharishi Ayurveda reconnect the individual's physiology of matter with its source in the physiology of consciousness. Some of the approaches do so by directly enlivening balance from the level of pure consciousness. Other approaches restore balance at the finest level of the physiology of matter—the level of the doshas—using highly individualized treatment and prevention programs based on a thorough understanding of diet, exercise, body natures, behavioral tendencies, and biological and seasonal rhythms. This integrated understanding of how to treat our physiology of consciousness and our physiology of matter promises to bring fulfillment to medicine's age-old dream to relieve mankind from disease and suffering.

Chapter 8

The Science of Veda

The steam rose off the ground on the hot plains of India. In the distance, the rumble of an occasional jet making its final approach to the Delhi airport could be heard.

Maharishi sat outside a small gazebo in the bright moonlight, in the company of an extraordinary group of Indian pandits and scholars. It was a scene that could well have taken place several millennia ago—except for a few Western scientists in the audience, the twentieth century hardly intruded.

"Man is not just a mass of cells," Maharishi explained. "In his simplest, most refined state of consciousness, man is the total potential of natural law, the field of pure potentiality, the Veda." The true meaning of the word Veda, he said, is not a collection of books from ancient India, as is commonly assumed by most Western and Eastern scholars. It is something entirely different. "Veda means knowledge," Maharishi said, "complete knowledge, inclusive of all life." He continued, "The Veda is present at every point in creation; it is the underlying unified field of pure knowledge, of pure consciousness, from which all diversity emerges."

I thought of the sharp contrast between this expanded vision of Vedic knowledge and our immature, localized vision of modern classical science, which does indeed see the body as a mass of cells that somehow has had life breathed into it. Certainly modern science has desired to embrace the essence of life—to touch both the very small and the very large. In this search for knowledge, however, it has adopted an objective methodology that obstructs its ability to see into the deepest subjective realms of consciousness. Maharishi Vedic Science and Technology offers a knowledge and methodology that brings fulfillment to modern science; it sees the human body as the microcosm of the macrocosm—the universe—in which all the dynamics of nature are expressed.

The Vedic Paradigm

What distinguishes the Vedic viewpoint from that of modern physics? Modern physics has grown to rely on the objective method of gaining knowledge, which has touched upon, but has not uncovered the true nature of the observer himself—the very consciousness of the scientist. Whole areas of vital knowledge concerning the subjective nature of consciousness have been neglected precisely because the objective approach could not reliably probe them.

Into the narrow intellectual atmosphere created by the dominance of modern science-based approaches, Maharishi has boldly introduced a new paradigm, the Vedic paradigm. This worldview restores the fundamental understanding that consciousness is the basic field of life. It is derived from Maharishi's revitalization of the profound wealth of Vedic wisdom. The manner in which he has brought this wisdom to light is of inestimable importance to mankind. He has taken a thoroughly modern and scientific angle to create a new science, his Vedic Science and Technology, which unifies the two polarities of the subjective and objective approaches to gaining knowledge. He has also encouraged scientists and scholars around the world to investigate, substantiate, and express Vedic wisdom using the terminology and technology of modern science.

When we say "natural law," we mean that intelligence which administers the whole universe, which right now is administering the functioning of our entire physiology, our heartbeat, our breathing, our brain wave activity, the activity of all the people on the earth, of the whole field of nature, and of the entire universe. This is natural law—it is an extraordinary intelligence, an infinite intelligence, which has infinite creativity and infinite organizing power. It is constantly and perpetually throughout time administering the evolution of the whole universe.

Both modern science and Maharishi Vedic Science describe the fundamental state of all the natural laws operating throughout the entire universe as the unified field of natural law—the basic, self-interacting, unlimited field of nature's intelligence—the single, universal source of all the orderli-ness in nature. The unified field is the level of the total intel-ligence of nature.

Not only is this field the basis of all natural law; it creates from within itself all the diverse laws of nature governing life at every level of the manifest universe. How does it do this? The unified field of natural law is not static—again, it is a lively, self-interacting field of intelligence. It interacts within itself, and the dynamics of its self-interaction give rise to a process of precise sequential unfoldment of the laws of nature.

In the Vedic paradigm, the unified field is therefore not only the source of matter, but also—because it is pure con-sciousness—the source of mind. It is the common source of mind and body, of subjective experience and material cre-ation. Consciousness is therefore the underlying field from which matter arises, as we have explained earlier. Further, the investigation of the unified field of natural law is not con-fined to intellectual analysis; this field can be directly experi-enced through the subjective technologies of consciousness Maharishi has brought to light from the Vedic literature.

Thus Maharishi Vedic Science describes the self-inter-acting dynamics of the unified field as the eternal dynamics of consciousness knowing itself. From this self-interaction within the unified field of pure consciousness, the laws of na-ture begin to unfold. As they unfold, they take form as the expressions of pure knowledge, known in Maharishi Vedic Science as the Veda. The same fundamental laws of nature described mathematically in the unified quantum field theories of modern physics are embodied in the structure of the Rik Veda, the most fundamental aspect of the Vedic literature.

Rik Veda is the first of the four principal Vedas; the other three are Sama Veda, Yajur-Veda, and Atharva Veda. The Vedic literature comprises these four, together with all the subsequent sections that constitute what Maharishi describes as the major "branches" and "limbs" of Vedic knowledge. The various texts of Ayurveda are a part of the body of knowledge. In Maharishi's explanation, Vedic literature displays the complete sequence of unfoldment of natural law from its source in pure consciousness, through all its increasingly more concrete expressions in every area of individual life—mind, body, and behavior—and to its fulfillment in all these areas and in the life of the entire universe.

Maharishi has referred to the Rik Veda as the Constitution of the Universe. We don't usually think of the universe as having a constitution. But every body of laws, whether man-made or nature's laws, is organized by some underlying, unifying principles. Just as the constitution of a nation represents the most fundamental level of national law and the basis of all the laws governing the nation, the Rik Veda, the Constitution of the Universe, represents the most fundamental level of natural law and the basis of all known laws of nature.

Maharishi defines the Constitution of the Universe as "the eternal, non-changing basis of natural law and the ultimate source of the order and harmony displayed throughout creation." This level of nature, he says, is lively in the intelligence of every grain of creation. There is a precise mathematical correspondence between the descriptions of the unified field of modern science and the field of pure consciousness. Most important, it is not only valuable to understand the Constitution of the Universe, but also to actually experience and enliven this level of nature's intelligence in our own minds, so that its total potential can be lived in our life.

Not only does the Vedic Paradigm bring new, unforeseen depth to the study of human physiology, it gives us the ability to reconnect individual life with its foundation in the unified field of natural law, so that life can be lived in accord with all the laws of nature.

The unified field is one single, universal field underlying—transcendental to—all existence. Yet within this transcendental field of unity exists the Rik Veda, the Constitution of the Universe, like a beautiful fabric containing innumerable permutations and patterns. Modern science calls these patterns "the laws of nature." In the Vedic paradigm, however, these laws or patterns are not seen as isolated material phenomena; on the contrary, they are woven into the fabric of pure consciousness itself.

The implications of the Vedic paradigm are far-reaching. They are found in every area of life. We have discussed at length the application in the field of health and medicine, as Maharishi Ayurveda. The theoretical basis of Maharishi Ayurveda is found in Maharishi Vedic Science and Technology, which includes a complete understanding of the relationship between mind and body.

The fundamental premise of Maharishi Vedic Science and Technology is that mind and body are both expressions of the laws of nature within one unified field, the unified field of pure consciousness. All aspects of physiology are studied in light of their emergence from, and connection to, the unified field of pure consciousness.

The Sounds of Nature's Intelligence

Maharishi Vedic Science and Technology covers the whole field of Veda, and its expression, the universe. It covers all knowledge about everything in the universe. As DNA is to the body, the Veda is to the universe. In this sense we can consider the Veda as "the physiology of the universe." Now we want to explore more deeply the physiology of the universe, the Veda itself, which, like DNA, underlies and creates all the expressed levels of manifest existence.

The sounds of the Veda arise from the "hum" of the vibration produced by the self-interacting dynamics of pure consciousness. This is what Maharishi refers to as "the language of nature," the "whisper" of the unified field of natural law to itself.

As the laws of nature unfold and eventually create all the material forms and phenomena of creation, they are displayed as *shruti*. Shruti refers to the sound value of the expressions of pure knowledge, Veda and the Vedic literature, as they unfold from within pure consciousness. Maharishi defines shruti as "vibrancy of intelligence in the form of sound generated by the self-referral dynamics of consciousness."

Maharishi describes the Vedas as "a beautiful, sequentially available script of nature in its own unmanifest state, eternally functioning within itself and, on that basis of self-interaction, creating the whole universe and governing it." And yet this simple and beautiful structure of natural law has been greatly misunderstood.

"The principal misunderstanding of the Vedas," Maharishi explains, "is that they are books or objects to be known or studied. The Vedas are *Apaurusheya*—that is, not created by individual minds, not even created by enlightened minds." Maharishi explains that the Sanskrit term Apaurusheya means "uncreated."

The Vedas, he says, are the "fundamental seeds of intelligence" from which all natural laws spring; they are the dynamic impulses of natural law which make up the fabric of the unified field. They existed before space and time, they are eternal and non-changing. Maharishi describes further, "They are nonindividual, existing on the level of the self-interacting dynamics of the unified field alone, the state of pure consciousness, pure awareness aware of itself."

If, however, we can speak of a "literature" of the Veda, doesn't that denote books and such? There are books known as the Vedas, which one can go to the library and read. If the Veda exists in consciousness, what are these books? How are they related to the Veda as the self-interacting dynamics of consciousness, and are they of any value to us in our desire to understand how natural law functions in the universe, particularly in the human body?

Describing the shruti aspect of the Veda, Maharishi explains that it refers to "those specific sounds that construct self-referral consciousness, which have been heard by the ancient seers in their own self-referral consciousness and are available to anyone at any time in one's own self-referral consciousness."

Maharishi traces the source of the Vedic tradition of knowledge all the way back to the dawn of creation, when great enlightened sages sat deep in meditation. Their awareness was so pure and refined that they heard the sounds of natural law, the whisper of the unified field to itself, in their own consciousness. They directly experienced the self-interacting dynamics of consciousness within their own highly enlightened awareness. These sages passed this wisdom down orally from one generation to the next; much later on these sounds were recorded and compiled by other great sages and teachers of the Vedic tradition. The Vedic literature is the record of these experiences of the enlightened.

Maharishi beautifully explains the connection of the Veda with human life. He says, "The knowledge of the unified field, Veda, is that self-whispering, self-interacting unified field which knows itself, which interacts with itself. We can very easily see this in the case of our own performance.

There is some area within us from where thoughts and emotions arise, from where all behavior comes out. That is the area of the unified field within us; that is the Veda within us."

Thus, the Veda is not something separate from us, something to be studied in a library. The Veda is within us, it is the true nature of our own consciousness. We want not only to understand the Veda intellectually; we want to know it on the level of direct experience as the self-interacting dynamics of our own consciousness. In fact, Maharishi's point is that this is the only way to really know the Veda.

If our nervous system is not refined enough to experience the self-referral dynamics of our own consciousness, then we cannot understand the Vedic literature; we cannot comprehend the essentials of nature's creativity. There is nothing to be gained from reading the Vedic literature in the waking state of consciousness; we will only become confused by the descriptions of nature's mechanics, which are expressed from the reality of higher states of consciousness. If, however, our nervous system is refined enough to have the experience of pure consciousness, then on that basis, as we grow toward higher states of consciousness, eventually we can discover and know the same eternal laws of nature's creativity that were experienced and known to the ancient Vedic sages.

Knowledge gained in this manner is not in any way "borrowed" knowledge; it is created afresh through the experience of higher states of consciousness. When one has attained higher states of consciousness, it becomes valuable to read and study intellectually the Vedic texts, as a way to confirm the level of experience and knowledge gained in those states.

Maharishi comments on another common misconception about the Veda: "The word 'Veda' has been badly promoted to be a religion of some people in the Himalayas, out of sight and out of mind. Veda is a very, very good friend of us all. We say 'Veda' because that is the word by which it likes to be called—'Veda' Veda is pure knowledge, and pure knowledge is organizing power."

Maharishi strongly emphasizes that the Veda is not confined to the people of one culture, nor is it a religion. Rather, it is a universal level of life that is the source of all knowledge in the universe, that is within each of us regardless of belief or religion. It is our most intimate level of consciousness.

The "technology" in Maharishi Vedic Science and Technology refers to specific, skillful uses of the sound value of the Veda to create, from the level of the self-interacting dynamics of consciousness, transformations on the outer, expressed level of life, including the concrete level of matter. Maharishi refers this to as Vedic engineering. The specific technologies used in Vedic engineering are the yagyas, which we have mentioned earlier. The Vedic literature contains the ultimate self-referral knowledge for human life: the Veda contains the knowledge of how to experience its own self-interacting dynamics, and thereby allow the human mind, body, and behavior to develop to enlightenment.

Role of Ayurveda in the Sequential
Unfoldment of Natural Law

This principal goal of Maharishi Ayurveda is to enliven the self-referral field of pure knowledge at the basis of the physiology, and on that basis to create balance in the body. As Maharishi explains,

> Ayurveda deals with the totality of life from the field of matter. It also prescribes the approach to regaining balance from the field of consciousness. It attends to the totality of the field of knowledge and to the field of the expression of knowledge, matter. Ayurveda deals with consciousness and matter. Working from both points of view, it recreates a very balanced personality. This is the approach of Ayurveda.

The knowledge of the Veda, Maharishi explains, handles the entire field of the science and technology of oneself. It covers infinite diversity and unity and puts them together in one package of knowledge. It is fortunate for us that the knowledge of Maharishi Ayurveda is available today to bring solutions to the many problems of humanity.

We can create balance and harmony not only in our lives, but in society. Over 50 studies, in fact, document this effect by showing that the practice of the TM technique and more advanced TM-Sidhi program, especially in a large group, can reduce crime and violence, improve the quality of life, and create peace in the world.

Chapter 9

The Vedic Scientist

Maharishi was fond of taking boat rides, whether on Lake Lucerne in Switzerland or Lake Tahoe in California.

Maharishi's lectures during these excursions have brought out some of the most profound and deep knowledge I have ever experienced. I remember one time when I gained perhaps my clearest understanding of Maharishi's description of the language of the Veda. This was during a boat ride with Maharishi in the spring of 1982, on the Rhine River near Boppard, Germany. On this occasion the physicist Dr. John Hagelin was present and the subject of discussion was the language of nature.

Maharishi explained that if we want to comprehend the Veda, then we must experience it in the language of the Veda itself. As he said, "The Veda must sing its own story; in its original script the Veda is just the whisper of the unified field to itself." Dr. Hagelin pointed out that a similar situation applies in physics: if we try to understand the quantum world from a classical perspective we fail to appreciate its full value;

we can gain only an approximation of that reality. In the classical realm we assume that matter and events are concrete, localized, and predictable.

In the quantum realm matter is neither solid nor static. It is only a condensation, or a concentrated manifestation of an underlying unmanifest quantum field. In order to understand the quantum world we must use the language of the quantum world. Only then, Dr. Hagelin explained, can we comprehend its complete subtlety and wholeness.

In a similar manner, Maharishi went on, if we want to properly understand and describe the Veda, we can do so only from the level of the experience of higher states of consciousness. We need to experience consciousness interacting with itself. This, Maharishi said, is the most profound language of nature—the Veda—which we come to know when we experience nature at its source.

Once we have the experience of higher states of consciousness, Maharishi continued, it is easier to understand waking state consciousness for what it truly is: a special, limited case of consciousness. Trying to understand intellectually the perspective of higher states of consciousness from the perspective of waking consciousness, without the experience of pure consciousness, may prove discouraging and create a sense of boundaries in the awareness rather growing freedom and fulfillment.

The discussion continued for several more hours. At the end, Maharishi summarized by explaining that each viewpoint is valid on its own level, yet the more comprehensive viewpoints give a fuller picture of nature. He referred to a key concept in the Vedic paradigm, "Knowledge is structured in consciousness." On one level, the meaning of this principle is expressed in a particular verse of Rik Veda: that the Veda—pure knowledge—exists in the transcendental field, pure consciousness, the Self. A corollary of that point is that our level of consciousness determines how deeply we can comprehend the Veda, and thus how much knowledge we can gain about the world. So far, our experience of the Veda, and thus our knowledge of the universe, has been limited because we have not had access to higher states of consciousness.

The Role of Experience

For over three hundred years, science has been in a quandary over the "problem" of mind and body. Why? Because it is a dilemma of waking state consciousness. In waking state consciousness we are confined to one viewpoint, which finds expression in one limited language of nature. It is indeed a very limited perspective whose language allows only the experience and understanding of separation between mind and body. The dilemma of waking state consciousness is the dilemma of modern science. In waking consciousness we cannot conceive of a state of pure subjectivity that underlies and creates all objective states of matter, including the body, except in the most superficial intellectual terms.

Only by transcending waking state consciousness, experiencing pure consciousness, and learning the new language of higher states of consciousness can we resolve this dilemma. As we know, pure consciousness is the unified state of knower, process of knowing, and known. From the perspective of this higher state of consciousness, mind and body are completely unified: there can be no separation between them, because the body is simply the objective, concrete expression of the same field of pure subjectivity that gives rise to the mind. The body is the physical form, the further expression of the self-interacting dynamics that creates the mind. Only by applying the technology of natural law, the Maharishi Technology of Consciousness, can we experience higher states of consciousness and use the full potential of our nervous system.

We know from neurophysiological research that different experiences can influence the structure and functioning of the brain. For example, when two groups of animals are raised in either a "rich" environment (containing many types of stimuli) or a "poor" environment (a standard small wire cage) the effects on the brain are significantly different. The animals living in the rich environment develop bigger and heavier brains (a thicker cerebral cortex) and exhibit increased amounts of a key biochemical communicator, acetylcholine. The most interesting difference, however, is a marked increase in interconnections among nerve cells in the animals living in an enriched environment.

The brain is never static or fixed. It is continually changing. With every experience neurotransmitter levels are increasing or decreasing, receptors are being replaced and neural connections are selectively strengthened or weakened. The structure and function of the brain is just a reflection of who we are. If we allow ourselves to become static and frozen in our personal development, locked into the waking state, then our once dynamic brain loses its dynamism and flexibility. If, on the other hand, we continually refine our neurophysiological functioning through the development of higher states of consciousness, then we will continue to unfold its latent potentialities.

As Maharishi has pointed out, it is a situation of "knock and the door will open"—DNA responds to the needs and the experiences presented by the environment. As we systematically and regularly experience transcendental consciousness, the brain becomes more coherent, more balanced. The results are clear from the myriad improvements seen in those who practice the Transcendental Meditation and more advanced TM-Sidhi program.

Vedic Perception

The Vedic literature is the record of the experiences of the ancient seers who thousands of years ago developed higher states of consciousness. The records of their experiences are in one sense similar to the records of experiments in modern scientific journals. They are repeatable results based on a systematic and repeatable experiential methodology, an inner technology of consciousness. Their object of inquiry was the laws of nature. Unlike modern scientific experiments, their methodology was subjective, their laboratory pure consciousness.

To have these experiences reliably and systematically, the first Vedic scientists, like any scientists, had to be experts in the appropriate technology, in this case the technology of consciousness. They had to refine the functioning of their nervous systems in order to be able to experience and develop higher states of consciousness. Maharishi explains that the Vedic seers perceived these laws of nature as reverberations of sound within their own consciousness. They passed down the knowledge they gained orally from one generation to the next, with the understanding that the actual meaning could be fathomed only if one first achieved higher states of consciousness. Precisely because the Vedic method of gaining knowledge depends on a fully developed nervous system, its main field of knowledge—the experience of the self-interacting dynamics of the Veda—long ago became inaccessible when the procedures to gain higher states of consciousness were not available.

The Vedic literature makes clear that this knowledge was available in its completeness in the ancient Vedic civilization. At that time many people regularly practiced these technologies and achieved higher states of consciousness: the knowledge of the Veda was the vibrant reality of their daily life.

However, Maharishi explains that after many generations living in the goal, the path to the goal—the technology of consciousness—was forgotten. Over the long course of history, as pure consciousness faded from the daily life of the people, the knowledge of the Veda became greatly misunderstood and misinterpreted. The situation was further complicated after the Vedic texts had been written down and eventually translated into other languages.

Without the experience of the self-interacting dynamics of consciousness, what remained were only the superficial outer trappings of knowledge. As Maharishi has commented, "The study of the Veda is not through the books of the Veda. . . . The study of the Veda is from what is inscribed in the pure consciousness of the individual student himself." Without the experience of pure consciousness, the student of the Veda could eat only the outer peel of the fruit of knowledge; the sweet fruit inside was unsuspected and therefore left untasted. In this situation, the fullness of life became cramped and daily life become full of suffering.

With Maharishi's restoration of the complete knowledge and experience of the Veda, these technologies have once again become widely available. Now it is possible for anyone to systematically and naturally experience pure consciousness as the ultimate basis of all subjective and objective states, and on that basis to become a Vedic scientist. With the experience of consciousness in its purest and most settled state, we become increasingly familiar with the fine fabrics of our own awareness—with the language of the unified field of natural law. We gain the ability to become Vedic physiologists—to examine directly the physiology of consciousness and to witness the physiology of the universe emerging from the vast sea of consciousness.

Maharishi beautifully describes the capability of a Vedic physiologist: "The Vedic physiologist can cognize the laws of nature directly within his own consciousness. They exist in their most concentrated form within the dynamics of consciousness. It is only necessary to be fully awake in the state of pure consciousness." Maharishi further explains the ensuing process of gaining knowledge of the laws of nature, based on one's having become fully awake in the state of pure consciousness:

> In the fully awake state of pure consciousness, the self-interacting dynamics of consciousness begin to reverberate within one's consciousness. The nature of the underlying threads of the fabric of consciousness begin to reveal themselves to themselves. The whole process is beautifully expressed in the Rik Veda, *Yojagara tam richa kamayante*— "He who is awake, the richas, the verses of the Veda, the impulses of natural law, seek him out." This is the prerequisite for gaining knowledge of the Veda.

The Vedic physiologist is thus able to directly perceive the innermost threads of consciousness as well as all the more manifest levels of the physiology of consciousness and the physiology of matter.

What would this experience be like? Maharishi gave a hint of what this Vedic perception would entail. He explained that in this highly developed state of enlightenment, the activity of each of the cells in our body should be apparent to us on the most refined level of hearing, as different voices in our consciousness. We would experience these impulses through the same consciousness—our Self—which is continually transforming itself into those impulses of sound and matter.

In this process, the body would become a kind of cinema cognized in terms of sound and vision as lively unity. If any impurity or abnormality happened to exist in our nervous system, then the impulses of consciousness (the sounds) would be out of harmony, or balance, with their "meaning" (that is, their precipitated form as matter). Then the highly discriminative ability of this most subtle perception would be lost.

In this case, the perception would be blurred. We might still hear the "hum" of the impulses of consciousness that structure the eyes, the tongue, the aggregate of cells—but we might not perceive the distinct value of the activity of each cell. But if our physiology were completely free of stress, pure and in balance, then the different values of all expressions of the Veda—the syllables and verses—would be distinctly perceived as the mechanics structuring the different values of physiology. As the refined perception characteristic of the highest states of consciousness developed, no aspect of natural law would be out of our comprehension. We would hear the whole verse and all of its parts, each syllable and at the same time the gaps between the syllables—the very mechanics of transformation within consciousness.

The true Vedic physiologists, from Maharishi's point of view, thus have access to the laws of nature within their own consciousness. They are able to cognize the Veda in terms of their own internal functioning. All this is possible because of the intimate relationship of the Veda with human physiology: one is merely a reflection of the other. The whole of the Veda is found embodied in the whole of human physiology.

Vedic scientists awaken within themselves the realization that located in the simplest form of awareness, their own Self, is the source of nature's creativity, the self-referral dynamics of pure consciousness. As we become Vedic Scientists we experience the self-interacting dynamics of consciousness within ourselves, and we come to know consciousness as the prime mover of life. We realize that Vedic Science is the science of our own consciousness: moving within itself, the wholeness of our consciousness creates the apparent diversity of the universe. Our own physiology is the physiology of the universe. Maharishi has described this ultimate realization of Vedic wisdom as embodied in the understanding that the total universe is contained in my Self: the Veda is all that there is, the Self is all that there is. This realization is expressed in the Vedic aphorism, *Aham Brahmasmi,* "I am the unbounded totality; I am everything."

Ramanyan in the Human Physiology

One of the greatest contributions to Maharishi's knowledge is the research of Dr. Tony Nader MD, PhD, who worked extensively with Maharishi to reveal the relationship between human physiology and the details of the Vedic literature. In his first book *Human Physiology: Expression of Veda and the Vedic Literature*, which we mentioned earlier, he shows that the order of Veda and the Vedic Literature is mirrored in the intrinsic order of our human physiology. In 1998 he received his weight in gold for this historic discovery of the complete expression of total Natural Law within the structure and function of human physiology, and in 2000 Maharishi honored him with the title of Maharaja Adhiraj Rajaraam, the first ruler of the Global Country of World Peace.

In his second book, *Ramayan in Human Physiology*, Dr. Nader unfolds even more detailed correlations focusing on the story of the Ramayan, a beloved of Indian culture. The Ramayan is at once a spiritual story about an avatar, an incarnation of God, and the story of perfect rulership and administration, as well as an epic hero tale that portrays the full range of human emotion. Dr. Nader's work reveals that the journey of the hero is an actual description of the neurophysiological mechanisms involved in the process of gaining enlightenment. Rather than describing physical transformations in today's scientific terms, the creators of these stories used the language of myth and poetry. The hero's final victory is the slaying of a demon, which symbolizes the removal of the stress in the body that supports destructive behavior. The significance of Dr. Nader's work is that the Ramayan can now be understand as a scientific description of the development of enlightenment in which we create coherent neural networks that enable us to realize our full mental potential.

Maharishi

In the Vedic tradition there have always been great individuals who have reached the very highest levels of perfection. Their knowledge and inspiration have always upheld the deep value of the Vedic wisdom. Their lives have determined the direction for generations to come. Today we are experiencing just such an event in human history. A new knowledge is emerging in this scientific age. The man, scientist and saint, who brought it forth, is Maharishi.

How was Maharishi able to bring to light the correct practice of this ancient technology of consciousness, which for centuries had been misunderstood? He has always given all credit for this revival of Vedic knowledge to his own teacher, Brahmananda Saraswati, known as Guru Dev, who was one of India's greatest teachers in the Vedic tradition. Late in his life Guru Dev accepted the position of the Shankaracharya of Jyotir Math in the Himalayas, a seat of leadership in the Vedic tradition that traces its descent from Shankara, who was responsible for an earlier complete revival of Vedic wisdom many centuries ago.

"The truth of Vedic wisdom is by its very nature independent of time and can therefore never be lost," Maharishi has written. Yet he describes how the original technology for developing higher states of consciousness was forgotten, not once, but many times throughout history, owing, he says, "to the long lapse of time." This, Maharishi explains, is "the tragedy of knowledge, the tragic fate that knowledge must meet at the hands of ignorance. It is inevitable, because the teaching comes from one level of consciousness and is received at quite a different level. The knowledge of unity must in time shatter on the hard rocks of ignorance."

The nervous system of an enlightened person must be keenly sensitive and extremely refined so that it can naturally and spontaneously experience the dynamics of the unified field of nature's intelligence. Since the time of the ancient Vedic rishis, there have been those who have experienced the unified field in its fullness, and gained enlightenment. At the times when the knowledge of the Veda had been temporarily lost to view, these were the great sages who again brought it to light from the Vedic literature in its full brilliance, to set the course of life to run in the most evolutionary direction to fulfill the high purpose of human existence.

Maharishi absorbed the complete experience and understanding of Vedic wisdom under his teacher's guidance and later began a formal, systematic restoration of it. Each new area of Vedic knowledge has been unfolded through Maharishi's research and penetrating vision into the Vedic literature, and he has inspired its integration with the latest advances in modern science and its formulation into practical educational programs that can be easily implemented everywhere.

By making available this knowledge and technology, Maharishi has given us the greatest resource on earth, the resource of the inner dynamics of consciousness. We must never lose the "memory" of our inner physiology of consciousness; we must never let our connection with it become weak. It is the source of all our creativity, all our success. It is the source of all the riches of nature.

There is a wonderful story Maharishi told. A saint crossing a river sees a scorpion in the water and bends down to pick it up and save it. The scorpion stings him and then falls back into the water. The saint tries to save it again, with the same result. After this happens several times the people nearby ask the saint, "Why are you trying to save that scorpion which is stinging you?" He answers, "Just as the nature of the scorpion is to sting, my nature is to save."

Maharishi's genius has extended to many areas of life, but his contribution to physiology and health is particularly significant, since physiology is that one area of life that bridges the divergent realms of subjectivity and objectivity, mind and body, consciousness and matter.

The knowledge of Maharishi Ayurveda is emerging in this scientific age as a practical technology of natural law to establish perfect health in the individual and society. What

Maharishi did when he brought out the Vedic literature and began teaching this extraordinary ancient science of physiology in the West was nothing less than the single most important scientific discovery of our age. It heralds the exploration of the greatest frontier of modern science, the understanding and practical application of the dynamics of consciousness.

Over the years Maharishi never stopped giving to the world his precious knowledge of his Vedic Science. Sometimes people have criticized this knowledge, but that did not stop Maharishi, who knew its true value. It is a knowledge that can and is transforming the world from problems and suffering to Heaven on Earth.

As Maharishi so beautifully explained,

> The Veda has been declaring throughout time: "Amrita-sya Putrah— Sons of Immortality." From the field of pure knowledge, the mortal has always been welcomed as the descendant of the Immortal. Modern science in its infancy, playing with the fine particles of nature, discovered the destructive potential of natural law, and has delivered total annihilation at the doorstep of human existence. Now it is high time for modern science in its present state of maturity to repay the debt it owes to life. Vedic Science offers the guiding principle. Vedic knowledge is emerging as the most profound science of life, and offers fulfillment to the human quest for perfection. This is the time for modern science to rise to fulfillment.

Maharishi Ayurveda and Food

In Maharishi Ayurveda, food is medicine. Maharishi Ayurveda has general recommendations for diet. To follow these recommendations, choose the diet of your dominant body nature. To determine your body type take the quiz at dharmaparenting.com.

Most Ideal Foods for Vata

The general guideline is that sweet, sour, salty, heavy, oily, and hot foods are best for Vatas. Pungent, bitter, astringent, light, dry, and cold foods are not good.

Best veggies: asparagus, beets, cucumbers, green beans, okra, radishes, sweet potatoes, turnips, carrots, and artichokes. Other vegetables may be eaten in moderation if cooked in ghee (clarified butter) or extra virgin olive oil, including a choice of peas, broccoli, cauliflower, zucchini, tomatoes, potatoes, leafy green vegetables, eggplants, orange and yellow peppers, mushrooms, and celery. Avoid or reduce cabbage or sprouts or raw vegetables.

Best spices: cardamom, cumin, ginger, cinnamon, salt, clove, basil, cilantro, fennel, nutmeg, oregano, sage, tarragon, thyme, a moderate amount of black pepper (also allspice, anise, asafetida, bay leaf, caraway, cardamom, juniper berry, licorice root, mace, marjoram, mustard).

Any organic dairy product is highly recommended. Milk is easier for Vatas to digest when heated. The warmth will also help to balance their Vata.

Favor rice, wheat, and oats (cooked, not dry). And reduce consumption of corn (fresh corn on the cob in season, however, is great), millet, barley, buckwheat and rye.

Favor sweet, well-ripened fruits such as apricots, plums, berries, melons, papayas, peaches, cherries, nectarines, and bananas. Also good are dates, figs, pineapples, mangoes, and avocados. If you have digestive problems, fruits are best eaten lightly cooked, stewed, or sautéed.

Generally all oils are good.

All sweeteners are acceptable.

Nuts and seeds are fine, especially almonds.

Vatas are usually very sensitive to gas-producing foods such as beans. Beans such as chickpeas, mung beans and tofu in small amounts are fine.

For nonvegetarians, favor fresh, organic chicken, turkey, fish, and eggs. Reduce or eliminate the consumption of red meat.

Most Ideal Foods for Pitta

The general guideline is that sweet, bitter, astringent, cold, heavy, and dry foods are best for Pittas. Pungent, sour, salty, and hot foods are not good.

Best veggies: asparagus, potatoes, sweet potatoes, leafy greens, broccoli, cauliflower, celery, okra, lettuce, green beans, peas, and zucchini. Also good are Brussels sprouts, cabbage, cucumbers mushrooms, sprouts, and sweet peppers. Avoid or reduce tomatoes, hot peppers, onions, garlic, and hot radishes.

All sweeteners may be taken in moderation, except for molasses and honey, which are heating to the system.

Dairy is helpful in balancing the heat of Pitta. Favor butter, ghee (clarified butter), milk, and ice cream. Since the sour taste can increase Pitta, sour or fermented products such as yogurt, sour cream, and cheese should be eaten sparingly.

Organic grains such as wheat, rice, barley, and oats are good. Reduce consumption of corn, rye, millet, and brown rice.

Sweet and ripe fruits like apples, grapes, melons, cherries, coconuts, avocados, mangoes, pineapples, oranges, and plums, are recommended. Also prunes, raisins, and figs are fine. Reduce or eliminate sour fruits such as grapefruit, cranberries, lemons, and persimmons.

Pittas need seasonings that are soothing and cooling. These include coriander, cilantro, cardamom, saffron, and fennel. Also turmeric, dill, fennel, and mint are fine. Spices such as ginger, black pepper, fenugreek, clove, salt, and mustard seed may be used sparingly. Completely avoid pungent hot spices such as chili peppers and cayenne.

Most nuts increase Pitta. Pumpkin seeds and sunflower seeds are alright.

Favor coconut, olive, and sunflower oils. Avoid or reduce almond, corn, safflower, and sesame oils.

Favor mung beans and chickpeas. Tofu and other soy products are alright.

For nonvegetarians, organic free range chicken and turkey are preferable. Red meat and seafood increase Pitta and should be avoided.

Most Ideal Foods for Kapha

The general guideline is that pungent, bitter, astringent, light, hot, and dry foods are best for Kaphas. Sweet, sour, salty, heavy, oily and cold foods are not good.

The vegetables recommended include asparagus, beets, broccoli, Brussels sprouts, cabbage, carrots, cauliflower, celery, eggplants, leafy greens, lettuce, mushrooms, okra, onions, peas, peppers, potatoes, spinach, and sprouts. Reduce consumption of vegetables such as sweet potatoes, tomatoes, cucumbers, and zucchini.

Favor skim milk. In general reduce dairy intake, which tends to increase Kapha. You can, however, add small amounts of ghee, whole milk, and eggs to the menu.

Honey (raw, unheated, and organic) is the only sweetener that helps balance Kapha. Avoid all other sweeteners.

Favor grains such as barley, corn, millet, buckwheat, and rye. Reduce intake of oats, rice, and wheat.

Beans of all types are good for Kaphas, except soybeans, tofu products, and kidney beans.

Fruits such as apples, apricots, cranberries, pears, and pomegranates are good. Avoid or reduce fruits like avocados, bananas, pineapples, oranges, peaches, coconuts, melons, dates, figs, grapefruits, grapes, mangoes, papayas, plums, and pineapples.

All spices except salt are good for Kapha. Pungent spices like ginger, pepper, and mustard seed are especially good. Reduce salt.

Except for pumpkin seeds and sunflower seeds, reduce the intake of all nuts and seeds.

Use small amounts of extra virgin olive oil, ghee, almond oil, corn oil, sunflower oil, or safflower oil.

For nonvegetarians, favor fresh, organic free range chicken and turkey. Limit or eliminate the consumption of red meat and seafood in general.

Ayurvedic Recommendations for Digestion

Ayurveda has dietary recommendations, but also gives recommendations to optimize digestion of our food.

Serve the main meal at noon when the digestive power is the highest.

Make sure you have given enough time to digest one meal before starting the next. This avoids the production of ama, or undigested food that is the source of disease in Ayurveda.

Sipping hot water throughout the day is especially good for Vatas.

Start the meal with a digestive aid, such as ginger juice and lemon.

Avoid cold water, especially with ice, before, during or after a meal since it reduces the flames of digestion (agni). Instead, serve small amounts of room-temperature or warm water with the meal. Ayurveda suggests that the stomach should be filled with one third liquids and one third solids, with one third left empty to allow for better digestion.

Always sit when eating and do not have other stimulation such as teelvision or phone conversations.

Conclude the meal with sitting quitely for five minutes.

Do not eat honey that has been cooked. Only add honey water that is not too hot (you can test it by placing your pinky finger into the hot water and making sure you don't feel any pain).

Notes and References

Chapter 1

Most of the original published research on the Transcendental Meditation and TM-Sidhi program is reprinted in *Scientific Research on Maharishi's Transcendental Meditation and TM-Sidhi Programme: Collected Papers*, Volumes 1-7. These are available through MUM Press (mumpress.edu). My original research includes several publications: Wallace, RK, Physiological Effects of Transcendental Meditation, 1970, *Science*, 167:1751-1754; Wallace, RK, et al., A Wakeful Hypometabolic Physiologic State, 1971, *American Journal of Physiology*, 221(3): 795-799; and Wallace, RK, et al., The Physiology of Meditation, 1972, *Scientific American*, 226(2): 84-90.

A complete analysis of the research is given in *The Neurophysiology of Enlightenment*, Dharma Press (2016). See Dr. Orme-Johnson's website TruthAboutTM.org for the most up-to-date review of research.

A description of the Transcendental Meditation technique and higher states of consciousness is given in Maharishi's books: *Science of Being and Art of Living: Transcendental*

Meditation, Plume, 2001 and *On the Bhagavad-Gita: A Translation and Commentary, Chapters 1-6*. MUM Press, 2015

Chapter 2

The passages quoted from Maharishi regarding DNA, RNA, and the transition from consciousness to matter at the beginning of this chapter are from *Inaugurating Maharishi Vedic University*. Maharishi's discussion of the tanmatras and mahabhutas is found in his translation and commentary on the Bhagavad-Gita, pp. 482-483.

Dr. Hagelin's two articles, from which his discussion of Panchamahabhuta theory in relation to modern physics is taken, are:

- Hagelin, JS, Is Consciousness the Unified Field? A Field Theorist's Perspective, *Modern Science and Vedic Science* 1987, 1(1): 29-87; and

- Hagelin, JS, Restructuring Physics from its Foundation in Light of Maharishi's Vedic Science, *Modern Science and Vedic Science* 1989, 3(1): 3-72.

Previous work on body types by Western researchers includes:

- Smith, HC, Psychometric Checks on Hypothesis Derived from Sheldon's Work on Physique and Temperament, *Journal of Personality*, 1949, 17: 310-320; and

- Friedman, M, *Type A Behavior and Your Heart* New York: Alfred A. Knopf, 1974.

Research on body types in Ayurveda includes:

- Schneider, RH, et al., (September 1985), Physiological and Psychological Correlates of Maharishi Ayurveda Psychosomatic Types, Paper presented at the Eighth World Congress of the International College of Psychosomatic Medicine, Chicago, IL;

- Singh, RH, et al., A Study of Tridosha as Neurohumors, 1980, *Journal of Research in Ayurveda and Siddha,* , 1(1): 1-20;

- Udupa, KN, *Stress and its Management by Yoga* Delhi: Motilal, Banarsidas, 1985;

- Prasher B et al., Whole genome expression and biochemical correlates of extreme constitutional types defined in Ayurveda. 2008, *J Transl Med*; 6:48;

- Mahalle NP et al. Association of constitutional type of Ayurveda with cardiovascular risk factors, inflammatory markers and insulin resistance. 2012, *J Ayurveda Integr Med;3(3):150-7.*

- Dey S, Pahwa P, Prakriti and its associations with metabolism, chronic diseases, and genotypes: Possibilities of newborn screening and a lifetime of personalized prevention. 2014, *J Ayurveda Integr Med*;5:15-24.

- Travis FT, Wallace RK, Dosha brain-types: A neural model of individual differences. 2015, *J Ayurveda Integr Med*;6:280-5.

Chapter 3

An excellent summary of the latest research on the microbiome can be found in *Brain Maker* by David Perlmutter, MD, Little Brown, 2015. See also wikipedia.

Chapter 4

Studies on biological rhythms include:

- Halberg, F, Implications of Biologic Rhythms for Clinical Practice, in Krieger, D. T., Hughes, J. C. (Eds.), *Neuroendocrinology* (Sunderland, MA: Sinauer Associates, 1980, pp. 109-119); and

- Halberg, F, et al., (August 15, 1973), Toward a Chronotherapy of Neoplasia: Tolerance of Treatment Depends on Host Rhythms, *Experientia* (Basel), 29: 909-934.

Chapter 5

The studies on Maharishi Ayurveda Bhasma Rasayana are:

- Nader, T., et al., (June 1987), Maharishi Ayurveda Bhasma Rasayana: Its Safety and Effectiveness in Animal Models of Diet-Induced Tissue Damage in Surgically Induced Brain Lesions and in Chemically Induced Cancer Lesions, Paper presented at the Twenty-Eighth Annual Meeting of the Society for Economic Botany, University of Illinois, Chicago, IL; and

- Nader, T, etal., (March 1987), Ayurvedic Rasayana Protects Against Kidney and Liver Damage in Rats Fed a Low-Lipotrope, High-Fat Diet, Federation Proceedings, 46(3): 959, Abstract 3747.

Dr. Hari Sharma's book is *Freedom from Disease: How to control Free Radicals, a major cause of aging and disease, A Scientist Rediscovers Prevention Oriented Natural Health Care: Maharishi Ayurveda* Toronto: Veda Publishing, 1993.

MAK and Cancer

- Patel, VK, et al., Reduction of Metastases of Lewis Lung Carcinoma by an Ayurvedic Food Supplement in Mice, 1990, *Nutrition Research*, 12: 51-61;

- Sharma, HM, et al., Antineoplastic Properties of Maharishi-4 Against DMBA-Induced Mammary Tumors in Rats, 1990, *Pharmacology, Biochemistry and Behavior*, 35: 767-773;

- Sharma, HM, et al., Antineoplastic Properties of Dietary Maharishi-4 and Maharishi Amrit Kalash Ayurvedic Food Supplements, 1990 *European Journal of Pharmacology*, 183: 193;

- Sharma, HM, et al., Anticarcinogenic Activity of an Ayurvedic Food Supplement, Proceedings of the 1988 Conference of the American Physiological Society/ American Society of Pharmacology and Experimental Therapeutics: 1988, *Abstracts* 86.1 and 86.2, A121;

- Prasad, KN, et al., Ayurvedic (Science of Life) Agents Induce Differentiation in Murine Neuroblastoma Cells in Culture, 1992, *Neuropharmacology*, 31(6): 599-607;

- Johnston, BH, et al., Chemotherapeutic Effects of an Ayurvedic Herbal Supplement on Mouse Papilloma, 1991, *The Pharmacologist*, 3: 39; and

- Wallace, RK, (June 1987), Maharishi Amrit Kalash and Its Effect on Natural Killer Cells, Paper presented at the *Twenty-Eighth Annual Meeting of the Society for Economic Botany*, University of Illinois, Chicago.

MAK and the Immune System

- Dileepan, KN, et al., Priming of Splenic Lymphocytes After Ingestion of an Ayurvedic Herbal Food Supplement: Evidence for an Immunomodulatory Effect, 1990, *Biochemical Archives*, 6:267-274;

- Patel, V, et al., (March 20, 1988), Enhancement of Lymphoproliferative Responses by Maharishi Amrit Kalash (MAK) in Rats, *Federation Proceedings*, 2(5), Abstract no. 4740; and

- Glaser J, et al., Improvement in Seasonal Respitory Allergy with an Ayurvedic Herbal Immunomodulator *J Ayurveda Health* 2015; 13,3

MAK and the Cardiovascular System

- Sharma, HM, et al.,. Maharishi Amrit Kalash (MAK) Prevents Human Platelet Aggregation, 1989, *Clinica & Terapia Cardiovascolare*, 8(3): 227-230.

MAK and Psychophysiological Well-Being

- Sharma, HM, et al., (January-March 1991), Effect of Maharishi Amrit Kalash on Brain Opioid Receptors and Neuropeptides, *Journal of Research and Education in Indian Medicine* 20(1): 1-8; and

- Hauser, T, et al., (November 14, 1988), Naturally Occurring Ligand Inhibits Binding of [3H]-Imipramine to High Affinity Receptors, Paper presented at the 18th *Annual Meeting of the Society for Neurosdence*, Toronto, Ontario, Canada, Abstract 99.19.

MAK and Free Radicals

- Niwa, Y, Effect of Maharishi 4 and Maharishi 5 on Inflammatory Mediators—With Special Reference to Their Free Radical Scavenging Effect, 1991, *Indian Journal of Clinical Practice*, 1(8): 23-27;

- Dwivedi, C, et al., Inhibitory Effects of Maharishi-4 and Maharishi-5 on Microsomal Lipid Peroxidation, 1991, *Pharmacology*, Biochemistry and Behavior, 39:649-652;

- Sharma, HM, et al., (October 6-11, 1991), Inhibition in Vitro of Human LDL Oxidation by Maharishi Amrit Kalash (M-4 & M-5), Maharishi Coffee Substitute (MCS) and Men's Rasayana (MR), Paper presented at the International Atherosclerosis Society, 9th International Symposium on Atherosclerosis, Rosemont, IL, Abstract 112;

- Panganamala, R. V., Sharma, H. M. (October 6-11, 1991), Antioxidant and Antiplatelet Properties of Maharishi Amrit Kalash (M-4) in Hypercholesterolemic Rabbits, Paper presented at the International Atherosclerosis Society, 9th International Symposium on Atherosclerosis, Rosemont, IL, *Abstracts* 110 and 111.

MAK and General Health

- Gelderloos, P, et al., Influence of Ayurvedic Herbal Preparation on Age Related Visual Discrimination, 1990, *International Journal of Psychosomatics*, 37(1-4): 25-29;

The National Cancer Institute studies are described by Barnard Sherman in "From Cancer Prevention to Life Extension: Research on Maharishi Amrit Kalash Proliferates," in the August 1991 issue of *MIU World*, p. 25.

A major study on the effects of aspirin is reported in The Steering Committee of the Physicians' Health Study Research Group—Preliminary Report (1988), Findings from the Aspirin Component of the Ongoing Physicians' Health Study, *New England Journal of Medicine*, 318(4): 262-264.

Studies on Spices:

- GreenMedInfo.com.
- NIH-listed human clinical trials on curcumin (http://clinicaltrials.gov/ct2/results?term=curcumin).
- http://www.who.int/mediacentre/factsheets/fs312/en/
- http://www.diabetes.org/diabetes-basics/diabetes-statistics/
- http://www.idf.org/diabetesatlas/5e/the-global-burden.

Chapter 6

Dr. Susumu Ohno's work includes:

- Ohno, S, Repeats of Base Oligomers as the Primordial Coding Sequences of the Primeval Earth and Their Vestiges in Modern Genes, 1984, *Journal of Molecular Evolution*, 20(3-4): 313-321; and
- Ohno, S, Ohno, M, The All Pervasive Principle of Repetitious Recurrence Governs Not Only Coding Sequence Construction But Also Human Endeavor in Musical Composition, 1986, *Immunogenetics*, 24(2): 71-78.

The research on nasal cycles and EEG is reported in: Wemtz, DA, et al., Alternating Cerebral Hemispheric Activity and the Lateralization of Autonomic Nervous Function, 1983, *Human Neurobiology*, 2: 39-43.

Further discussion of left-right brain functioning is found in Gazzaniga, M. S., *The Bisected Brain* New York: Appleton-Century-Crofts, 1970.

Other research on the approaches of Maharishi Ayurveda, particularly Maharishi Panchakarma purification procedures, includes:

- Schneider, RH, et al., Health Promotion with a Traditional System of Natural Health Care: Maharishi Ayurveda, 1990, *Journal of Social Behavior and Personality*, 5(3): 1-27;

- Smith, D. E., Stevens, M. M. Pilot Project: The Effects of a Sesame Oil Mouth Rinse on the Number of Oral Bacteria Colony Types, Paper presented at the 1988, Third Annual Scientific Meeting of the College of Health Professions, Wichita State University;

- Salerno, JM, Smith, DE, The Use of Sesame Oil and Other Vegetable Oils in the Inhibition of Human Colon Cancer Cells in Vitro, 1991, *Anticancer Research*, 11: 209-216;

- Smith, DE, Salerno, JM, Selective Growth Inhibition of Human Malignant Melanoma Cell Line by Sesame Oil in Vitro, 1992, *Prostaglandins, Leukotrienes, and Essential Fatty Acids*, 46:145-150;

- Bauhofer, U. et al., Application of Maharishi Ayurveda in Infection with the Human Immune Deficiency

Virus (HIV)—Case Reports, Presented at the 1988, *Fourth International Conference on AIDS*, Stockholm, Sweden; and

- Waldschutz, R, Physiological and Psychological Changes Associated with Ayurvedic Purification Treatment, 1988, *Erfahrungsheilkunde—Acta Medico Empirica—Zeitschrift fur die drztliche Praxis*, 2: 720-729.

Chapter 7

Maharishi's discussion of balance and imbalance mediated by the intellect is found in *Life Supported by Natural Law*. The quotations from Maharishi about Veda as the script of nature are from *Inaugurating Maharishi Vedic University*.

The study on the effect of primordial sound on cancer cells is:

- Stephens, RE, et al., Effect of Different Sounds on Growth of Human Cancer Cell Lines in Vitro, 1992, *Federation Proceedings*, 6(5): A1934 (Abstract).

The research on Veda and the Vedic literature is:

- *Human Physiology: Expression of Veda and the Vedic Literature* by by Maharaja Adhiraj Rajaraam, Dr. Tony Nader, Maharishi Vedic University Press 2001

Chapter 8

Maharishi's initial statements on Veda and the mass of cells were made during a lecture in India in 1986; a similar discussion appears in the first edition (1974) of the Maharishi International University catalog. Maharishi's definitions of his

Vedic Science have appeared in "Maharishi's Vedic Science: Definition and Scope," in the Manifesto of the Natural Law Party, England, 1992. The discussion of the sequential unfoldment of natural law and the Vedic literature in Maharishi's Vedic Science is based on that found in several sources, including: *Maharishi's Absolute Theory of Government: Automation in Administration, Inaugurating Maharishi Vedic University, Life Supported by Natural Law, and Maharishi Vedic University Bulletin* (1985).

An excellent discussion of the unfoldment of Vedic literature in Maharishi's Vedic Science is given by Dr. Michael C. Dillbeck (1988) in The Mechanics of Individual Intelligence Arising from the Field of Cosmic Intelligence—The Cosmic Psyche, *Modern Science and Vedic Science*, 2(3); 245-278. Maharishi's concluding statements about Maharishi Ayurveda, pulse diagnosis, and the Vedic literature were made during a lecture in December 1992 in Vlodrop, the Netherlands.

Chapter 9

Maharishi's discussion of DNA is from a lecture in India in 1986, *Inaugurating Maharishi Vedic University* and *Maharishi's Absolute Theory of Government*.

The research on experience and the brain includes:

- Rosenzweig, MR, et al., Brain Changes in Response to Experience, 1972, *Scientific American*, 226: 22-29; and

- Diamond, C.,, et al., Effects of Environment on Morphology of Rat Cerebral Cortex and Hippocampus, 1976, *Journal of Neurobiology*, 1: 75-86.

The research on the Ramanayan is: *Ramanyan in the Physiology: Discovery of the Eternal Reality of the Ramanyan in the Structure and Function of Human Physiology*, by Maharaja Adhiraj Rajaraam, Dr. Tony Nader, MUM Press, 2011

Maharishi's comments on the loss and revival of knowledge are greatly elaborated in the preface to his book *On the Bhagavad-Gita: A Translation and Commentary, Chapters 1-6*, p. 16.

Other points of Maharishi's discussion are taken from Maharishi's commentary on the Bhagavad-Gita, noted above; *Maharishi Mahesh Yogi, Thirty Years Around the World: Dawn of the Age of Enlightenment*, Vol. 1, 1957-1964; *Inaugurating Maharishi Vedic University*, and Maharishi's introductory statements in the journal *Modern Science and Vedic Science*, pp. i-ii.

Related Websites and Books

TM.org
TruthAboutTM.org
MUM.edu
DavidLynchFoundation.org
DharmaParenting.com
DharmaPublications.com

An Introduction to Transcendental Meditation: Improve Your Brain Functioning, Create Ideal Health, and Gain Enlightenment Naturally, Easily, Effortlessly by Robert Keith Wallace, PhD, and Lincoln Akin Norton, Dharma Publications, 2016

Transcendental Meditation: A Scientist's Journey to Happiness, Health, and Peace, Adapted and Updated from The Physiology of Consciousness: Part 1 by Robert Keith Wallace, PhD, Dharma Publications, 2016

The Neurophysiology of Enlightenment: How the Transcendental Meditation and TM-Sidhi Program Transform the Functioning of the Human Body, Adapted and Updated from The Physiology of Consciousness: Part 2 by Robert Keith Wallace, PhD, Dharma Publications, 2016

Transcendence: Healing and Transformation through Transcendental Meditation by Norman Rosenthal, Tarcher/Penguin 2011

Transcendental Meditation: Revised and Updated by Robert Roth, Primus, 1994

Science of Being and Art of Living: Transcendental Meditation by Maharishi Mahesh Yogi, Plume, 2001

Catching the Big Fish: Meditation, Consciousness, and Creativity by David Lynch, Tarcher/Penguin, 2007

Dharma Parenting: Understand Your Child's Brilliant Brain for Greater Happiness, Health, Success, and Fulfillment by Robert Keith Wallace PhD, and Fredrick Travis PhD, Tarcher/Penguin, 2016

Dharma Health and Beauty: A User-Friendly Introduction to Ayurveda, Book One of the Smith Family Saga by Samantha Wallace with Robert Keith Wallace, PhD, Dharma Publications, 2016

The Transcendental Meditation Technique and The Journey of Enlightenment by Ann Purcell, Dragon Publishing Group, 2015

Maharishi Mahesh Yogi and His Gift to the World by William F. Sands, PhD, MUM Press, 2013

Acknowledgments

I would like to acknowledge both Susan Shatkin and my wife, Samantha, for their enormous help in editing. I would also like to thank Allen Cobb for his help in preparing this book, Fran Clark for proofreading, and George Foster for his excellent cover design.

About the Author

ROBERT KEITH WALLACE is a pioneering researcher on the physiology of consciousness. His work has inspired hundreds of studies on the benefits of meditation and other mind-body techniques. Dr. Wallace's findings have been published in Science, American Journal of Physiology, and Scientific American. He received his BS in physics and his PhD in physiology from UCLA, and he conducted postgraduate research at Harvard University. Dr. Wallace is founding president and member of the board of trustees of Maharishi University of Management (MUM) in Fairfield, Iowa, He is Co-Dean of the College of Perfect Health and Professor and Chairman of the Department of Physiology and Health.

Index

K

kapha 18, 19, 21, 23, 24, 26, 27, 29, 32, 39, 47, 120, 121

L

lifestyle medicine 3, 4
Lynch, David 136

M

mahabhutas 14, 15, 16
Maharishi 1, 2, 4, 5, 8, 11, 13, 14, 15, 16, 17, 18, 19, 20, 21, 23, 24, 28, 29, 30,
    31, 32, 33, 37, 39, 40, 43, 45, 46, 47, 48, 51, 52, 53, 54, 55, 56, 59, 62, 64,
    67, 68, 70, 71, 73, 74, 75, 77, 78, 79, 80, 81, 83, 84, 85, 86, 87, 89, 90, 91,
    92, 93, 94, 95, 96, 97, 98, 99, 100, 101, 102, 104, 105, 106, 107, 108, 109,
    110, 111, 112, 113, 114, 115, 117, 136
Maharishi Amrit Kalash 53, 54, 55, 56
Maharishi Ayurveda 1, 2, 4, 5, 11, 14, 17, 18, 19, 20, 23, 24, 28, 29, 30, 31, 32,
    33, 37, 39, 40, 43, 45, 46, 47, 48, 51, 52, 55, 59, 62, 64, 67, 68, 70, 71, 73,
    74, 75, 77, 79, 80, 81, 83, 84, 85, 87, 94, 100, 114, 117
Maharishi Ayurveda Bhasma Rasayana 52
Maharishi Colleges of Perfect Health 8
Maharishi Health Centers 8
Maharishi Jyotish 84, 85
Maharishi's Vedic Science 15, 16, 84, 90, 91, 92, 94, 95, 99
Maharishi's Vedic Science and Technology 15, 16, 90, 94, 95, 99
medicinal plants 4, 51, 53, 58, 62, 64, 65
microbiome 36, 41

N

Nader, Tony 53, 83, 111
nadi vigyan 19
natural health 2, 3
natural law 12, 13, 17, 68, 69, 79, 80, 84, 85, 86, 89, 91, 92, 93, 94, 95, 96, 97,
    104, 108, 109, 114, 115

O

ojas 41

P

panchakarma 73, 74, 75